So You're Going Bald!

So You're Going Bald!

Julius Sharpe

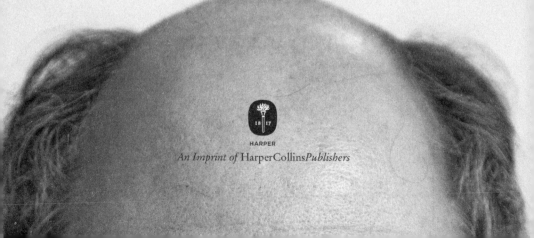

HARPER

An Imprint of HarperCollins*Publishers*

Images on page 13 courtesy of FBI (combo photo) and Sherburne County Sheriff's Office (bottom); images on pages 15–16, 36, 53, 134, 152, 154–156, 212, and 216 courtesy of the author; images on pages 47 and 64–68 courtesy of Charlie Hankin; images on pages 55–58 courtesy of Eli Green; image on page 74 courtesy of Charles C. Thomas, Publisher, Ltd., Springfield, Illinois; images on page 76 courtesy of Alila Medical Media (top) and Charles C. Thomas, Publisher, Ltd. (bottom); image on page 143 courtesy of Alec Sulkin; images on page 190 courtesy of MB Pictures/Shutterstock.

HarperCollins books may be purchased for educational, business, or sales promotional use. For information, please email the Special Markets Department at SPsales@harper collins.com.

FIRST EDITION

Designed by Nancy Singer

Library of Congress Cataloging-in-Publication Data has been applied for.

ISBN 978-0-06-285938-9

19 20 21 22 23　LSC　10 9 8 7 6 5 4 3 2 1

To Vin Diesel

"Adversity is the first path to truth."

—*Lord Byron*

"Damaged people are dangerous. They know they can survive."

—*Josephine Hart*

"Holy shit, I'm going bald! What the fuck?!"

—*You*

Contents

Preface

Baldness.

It's every man's greatest fear—you'll lose your hair, it will ruin your looks and destroy your life. It seems insane that it's 2019 and baldness is still legal, yet here we are.

If you're holding this book, it's undoubtedly because you're losing hair and you're freaking out. Your head, once a great source of pride and joy, now looks like the landing pad for a drone. You've long thought of bald people as solitary, pathetic testicles, and the last thing you ever imagined is you would become one yourself. But now it's happening and you're terrified, you're ashamed, and you don't know what to do.

But the one thing you're not is . . . alone. I mean, sure, you're currently by yourself reading, and the person you think of as your "best friend" would be shocked to hear that. But you're not alone in the larger, universal sense.

More than 40 million American men are bald, yet if you walk into any bookstore, *there isn't even a Bald section.* Wait—it gets worse: there isn't even a *single* book about going bald. The entire collected knowledge of the history of mankind has zero advice to offer the bald man. Until now.

Look around you: Every single other book in this store is for people with hair. Sure, there are thousands of books about dating, losing weight, and getting rich, but none of them will work for you because *there's nothing on top of your head.* In fact, the entire world is built for people with hair. Us balds are expected to be thankful just scurrying around in our emotional gulag until we're cremated along with all the unwanted cats.

Well, no more—what you are holding in your hands is more precious than gold, or, depending on when you're reading this, Bitcoin. *So You're Going Bald!* is the first-ever book to teach bald and balding men how to succeed in the world. It's part educational, part inspirational, and in an emergency, it's even edible. It's a rollicking "losing-of-hair memoir," plus a one-stop guide for bald men and the people who claim to love them. By reading it, you can regain everything you used to have: hopes, dreams, passion, excitement. (Basically everything *except* hair.) *So You're Going Bald!* is your new Bible, so you can throw that old Bible away!

And you don't even have to be bald to read it! In fact, if you have hair, this book may be even *more* important. Just as *Angela's Ashes* makes you think, "My life isn't so bad—at least I'm not an Irish child being beaten," or *Fifty Shades of Grey* makes you think, "I'm glad a prominent businessman isn't choking me during sex," *So You're Going Bald!* will inspire gratitude. If you're not bald, whatever you're dealing with in life—poverty, illness, the feeling you own all the wrong shirts—reading this book will show you that anything is surmountable because you have hair.

But most people reading this *are* bald. And the worst thing about baldness—even more than the panic and desperation—is that there's basically no honest information about what's happening to you and what you can do about it.

Well, for once, you're about to get a straight answer to all your questions about losing your hair and, toward the end, you'll also get a ten-minute recipe for salmon. I'm not gonna sugarcoat it, my advice or the salmon. It's not going to be easy (baldness—the salmon is a cinch), but when it's over, you will emerge from hair loss a better person, with a quick, antioxidant-rich meal for one.

I will explain your emotional plight and how to overcome it. I will review the current solutions to hair loss and offer real-world recommendations based on my experience. I will tell you how to market yourself to get dates, and what to do on those dates. I will teach you definitively who killed JFK and why. I will instruct you how to be bald at work. I will reveal why God took your hair back. You'll learn all the tips and tricks you need to survive as a bald man, and finally, I will walk you through how to prepare for death and help you plan your eventual funeral. After that, you're on your own.

First and most important, I want to assure you: Even though you're bald, you will be able to have a normal life.

I know it doesn't seem that way. You look around, and it seems like every guy holding hands with a gal has a man bun. Everyone dry humping on the docks has a beautiful pompadour. Every teacup ride is "Hair Only." Your bald head on Tinder might as well be a "swipe left" tattoo. ("Left" is when you don't want someone, right? I'm married and my wife is reading this, so I definitely have no idea how Tinder works, nor do I want to! Endless biweekly monogamous lovemaking is far superior to casual sex with young, polyethnic strangers!)

I understand how everything—job prospects, love, fun, happiness—feels like it's going down the shower drain with your hair, and maybe even your pee, depending on your attitude toward that type of thing. I understand the sleepless nights, the long days, the mornings that actually seem like the right amount of time. I understand the agony you feel looking in the mirror. I understand the excruciating top-of-head sunburns.

I understand all this because I, Julius Sharpe, am bald.

That's right. I was once exactly where you are: I had just graduated college with a 2.3 average, I owned a Kia Rio (finished in Ice Wine, S trim), and I was about to seek my fame and fortune in Delaware. Then, my hair went bye-bye and it seemed like my life was going to be over before it had really gotten started.

But now, I've completed my own courageous journey through baldness, so I can teach you how bald men can be successful in work, play, love, and even fantasy sports! Hairless and broke at thirty, I've successfully navigated hair loss to become the rarest thing in Hollywood: a middle-aged Jewish writer. I went from losing my hair to living in a 1,500-square-foot house in a part of Los Angeles that hasn't burned down yet. I own two (!) bicycles. I have a job where there are free peanuts in the kitchen, and I have almost $7,000 saved toward retirement.

If you had told me any of this was possible when I started going bald, I would have laughed in your face. Then, if no one was around, I would have kicked you really hard, then shoved you down a flight of stairs. Then, panicked over what I had just done, I would have cleaned up all the blood, rolled you in a carpet, and buried your rugbody in a perfect murder ravine I've made a mental note of several times while driving back from Las Vegas. Then, I would have put a crossword puzzle in the local paper with clues to taunt the cops.

But it's true, your life isn't over—not if you recalibrate your expectations, swallow a dose of humility, and change your approach in the bedroom, the boardroom, and even the bathroom. I'll walk you through new tactics for dating, conversation, grooming, and health. These techniques have been honed for centuries, lovingly handed down to me by generations of bald shamans and medicine men, and now I'm selling them to you.

By following my simple advice, you *can* achieve success, especially if you're living in Alabama or the Philippines, where housing is very cheap! You're going to have to read, which is harder than watching TV, but by the end you'll feel something you haven't felt for a long time: hope.

Whether you're eighteen and just noticed your first hair in the drain, or you're a hundred and eight and someone put this book in your hands several hours ago then left, there's no one better than me to help you. For starters, I recently passed my "Hairquator," the date past which you've been bald for longer than you've had hair. It's been so long, I've forgotten what it's even like to have hair. It's been so long, *I'm now bald in my dreams.*

You need answers, and I've got 'em. I'm the older bald man you've long wished would take a nonsexual interest in you. I'm here to give you the tough love you need, the pat on the back, the shot in the arm, the weird, overly long massage of the foot. Just as Khloé Kardashian nursed Lamar Odom back to health so he could leave her again, I hope to get *you* back on *your* feet, so one day you'll see me in the street, whisper "Thank you," then knee me in the balls. Together, maybe we can't beat baldness, but at the very least we can take all these jerks with hair down a peg.

You're probably thinking, "Okay, honey-tongued stranger. I'll listen to what you have to say. What do I have to lose? I'm shitting anyway." That's a great attitude and something to remember throughout this book: you're shitting anyway. It's this, or refresh your emails, and I know no one is emailing you, because you're fucking bald.

Are you ready? Your journey to a better life begins right now! Hold on to your hat! (By the way, you're going to need hats. A lot of them.) Hair we go!

Julius Safran Sharpe
Irkutsk, Siberia
December 25, 2018

So You're Going Bald!

1

What the Fuck Is Happening to Me?

Every bald man knows the horrific cycle: the realization, the panicked denial, followed by the endless spiraling anxiety.

From the first time there is an unusual amount of hair on a pillow, stuck to the soap, or tangled in a hairbrush, you've asked yourself the same question over and over, with increasing panic: *What the fuck is happening to me?*

Through compulsive examination, you've talked yourself into and out of the worst-case scenario thousands of times a day. "I'm going bald!" "It's nothing, I'm being crazy!" "That's an insane amount of hair to lose!" "That's normal! Everyone loses hair!"

You've examined your head morning, noon, and night, under every different kind of light, in mirrors, windows, and via the selfie thing on your phone. You've spent hours frantically obsessing: "Is that patch of skin a bald spot? Is it shrinking? Growing? Am I losing my hair, my mind, or both?!"

I've been where you are. I've googled surgeries, I've googled drugs, I've googled weird remedies. I've googled

"Googling weird drug surgery remedies." Like you, I've held a mirror in front of my head and a mirror behind it, losing myself in an infinite M. C. Escher vortex of my own baldness. Like you, I've set camera self-timers, then sprinted across the room, trying to find the one magic angle that could create a nonpathetic dating profile picture. Like you, I've spent thousands of hours scrolling through insane message boards to learn how the hell celebrities are "curing" their baldness. And, like you, I've wasted an enormous portion of my life trying to learn about baldness, combat baldness, or drinking to forget about baldness.

And occasionally, I've found, tequila works and you're able to have a few blissful moments without manic concern.

Then, someone on Instagram posts a picture of you at a party where you thought you were having a good time, and you look like a human tampon applicator. And the cycle begins again: more hysteria, more googling, more self-loathing, with even more intensity. I destroyed half my twenties and most of my thirties with this spiral, just like you. When I should have been out with my cool, gender-fluid friends eating avocado toast and planking, I was staring at my scalp as it vanished into thin hair.

When you're balding, it dominates your life from the moment you wake up to the moment you go to bed. You try to be normal at school or work but your mind races with questions all day. "What is going to happen to me? Can I still find happiness? Will I ever be in a relationship? Is everyone noticing? Is a cure coming? Is the cure here, but secret? Could I steal Sheila's baby and harvest its hair for donor plugs? Can I purchase human follicles on the dark web? How come Kim Jung Un, Chewbacca, and Tom Brady all get to have hair while I go bald?"

I never admitted to anyone how obsessed I was about my hairline, and how ashamed I felt about being obsessed. I was missing work, exhausted from not sleeping, and wearing a weird derby hat everywhere. Everyone assumed I was a severe heroin addict, not realizing I was simply just a desperate, alcoholic bald guy.

As a former astrophysics minor with a C-minus average, I couldn't stop fixating on how my baldness was sending me down a parallel universe. In one universe, I continued to have hair and lead an amazing "real" life. I had a great job, lots of money, a cool car, and just the right amount of sex. (Three times a week? Is that a lot? I mean, it sounds like a lot. Or am I a nerd and that's, like, nothing? Okay, I'd have sex fifteen times a week, you judgmental nympho!)

But this was not my real life. By some cruel twist of fate I was stuck in *this* universe instead, the one where I was going bald. I had started doing stand-up comedy three years prior (with a giant head of hair) and things were going well. I was making a couple hundred bucks a weekend and after shows I would often make out with desperate women from Long Island. Louis C.K. once told me I was funny, back before we all loved him, then hated him.

Then, hairs on the pillow destroyed my confidence. My performing career stalled out and I worked a series of dead-end jobs. Now *I* was the desperate one from Long Island. Women made excuses why we couldn't go out, never stating the obvious: They simply didn't want to look at me. Meanwhile, everyone I knew seemed to be finding the love of their lives. I was invited to fifteen weddings and always seated at the bald table—as though bald guys need to know more bald guys! I knew all that stood between me and a better life was hair, but I had no way to get it.

I was convinced there must be some secret information or cure I wasn't privy to and if I simply googled hard enough, I could find it and end this nightmare. I became a forensic investigator of celebrity hairlines, hoping to crack the case. No celebrity ever says, "I was balding. Here's what I had done." So either no celebrity has ever been bald (unlikely) or there's a whole world of classified tonsorial knowledge that we balding nobodies can't access.

Why won't these famous people—many of whom were obviously balding at some point then "miraculously" cured—admit what's happened and what they've done? They're scared. But why? Why is there more shame and secrecy around baldness in our society than anything else?

Celebrities will come clean about anything—addiction, infidelity, cheating at the Tour de France, human trafficking—anything *except* for one thing: how they got their hair back. Therefore, baldness must be the worst thing in the world! And these are celebrities, morons for whom everything has gone right! I'm no one! You're no one! What the hell are *we* supposed to do?

I've learned through hard-won experience: You can either sit around waiting for John Travolta to reveal the one, single, giant obvious secret he's hiding from everyone (his baldness? —it's his baldness, right?), or you can take control of your life.

Be real with yourself. If you think you're going bald, you *are* going bald. I've never met anyone who was losing a ton of hair, thought they were going bald, then realized they were just standing in the wrong light for fifteen years. The sooner you accept it, the sooner you can stop obsessing and start doing something about it.

My anguish was private, and I've made it my mission that no cue ball will suffer alone ever again. You may be going bald, but I'm going to make damn sure it doesn't destroy your life like it almost did mine.

Why Are You Going Bald?

I'll spare you the technical medical explanation, but as simply put in the March 2001 issue of the *Journal of Investigative Dermatology*, the polymorphism of your androgen receptor genes is overly sensitive to the presence of androgen dihydrotestosterone, leading to a higher incidence of shorter triplet repeat haplotypes. In other words, you have too much testosterone, and it's making you so horny it's blowing the hair off your head.

Okay, but *why* is the polymorphism of your androgen receptor genes overly sensitive to the presence of androgen dihydrotestosterone, leading to a higher incidence of shorter triplet repeat haplotypes?

Sadly, you inherited this genetic shit sandwich because one or both of your grandfathers was also a super horny bald weirdo. And *their* grandfathers were super horny, too, and *their* grandfathers were super horny, all the way back to some four-foot-six bald horn-dog with wooden teeth who never once showered and thought the earth was flat. Ironically, testosterone—the very same substance that drove them to procreate and eventually produce *you*—is ruining *your* chances at procreation. Ha-ha, good one, universe.

But don't feel bad for these hairless past-people just because they didn't have Netflix and they all died of the sniffles. Your ancestors had it easy. They got to drink at breakfast, and not just on vacation. And they lived in a time before dating, when you just married whichever cousin was standing next to you. However, *you* have to date. And you're not even really allowed to date one of your cousins, which really sucks, especially if you have hot cousins. Lack of cousin-dating is maybe the single greatest scourge facing the bald man today. Ah, to be alive in the 1600s, when your mom's brother's daughter was fair game, and a viable career was a ten-year global expedition for cinnamon.

So What Should I Do?

Well, the first and most important thing you need to do is take a deep breath. Inhale. Great. Exhale. Great. Inhale. Great. Exhale. Great. Get really, really calm. Perfect.

Now . . . PANIC. See red. Let raw terror and unbridled desperation fill your soul and hurl you into a boundless hysteria. It's not going to be okay! Anyone who says it's going to be okay is a liar. That's why just as a group of crows is called a "murder," a group of bald men is called a "suicide."

Are you hyperventilating now? Awesome. Really feel yourself unravel.

What the hell—you're a young man! You probably just got out of school, for the first time in your life you have no homework, you're ready to make your way in the world, and then . . . *the fucking top of your head falls off.* I mean, if God exists, how do you explain baldness? Or diarrhea?

(NOTE: Later, I will definitively solve the problem of God, so you'll never have to worry about it again. I'll leave diarrhea to the priests and rabbis.)

Hair becomes the former lover who's doing better without you. You see it partying with other men at clubs and restaurants looking lusher, thicker, and somehow happier than you remember. It's forgotten you even exist and is having the time of its life. And most maddeningly, it's the most committed to the people who treat it the worst! Like Jared Leto, dyeing it green or purple, just for kicks! Risking damage to those precious follicles, so awash in hirsute beauty, confident no matter what he does to them, they'll never leave. Leto can't even appreciate what he has. If I had Jared Leto's hair, I would stroke it, kiss it—heck, I'd buy it ice creams!

But you are not Jared Leto (unless you *are* Jared Leto and you're reading the wrong book), so there is one foolproof thing you can do to end the pain: Close your eyes and jump off a roof.

Does that feel better? I'm guessing no.

And that's how you learn the first lesson of baldness. The problem of being bald pales in comparison to severely broken bones and potentially never walking again. This is a technique I use all the time called "analysis by paralysis": A greater, more pressing problem will always distract you from a smaller one. Anytime you feel stress or that the world is closing in, simply grab a live power line or drive your car off a bridge. You'll feel better because you feel worse.

I could tell you that your life is going to improve, and that baldness is a mere bump in the road. But it's not. Baldness *is* the road and it's gonna tear your ass up. Your entire self-image will need to be recalibrated. How you see yourself and how others see you will never be the same.

The most immediate and life-shattering change is that baldness adds thirty years. The person you thought you are is now dead and replaced with a version of you that looks like an old baby or a young corpse. No one will take you seriously again. No manager has ever said, "Hey, let's give that giant, elderly baby more responsibility and a raise!" even if you're wearing a cute onesie.

Now, on top of everything else, you're not just fighting the stigma of being bald; you're fighting the stigma of being old, which sucks because you're not old!

If you *are* old, please skip the following paragraphs and rejoin us after the asterisks.

Everyone hates the elderly, and with good reason. They're super annoying. They walk and drive too slow, their butts aren't cute at all, and their breath absolutely reeks of shit and death. They can barely eat anything, then they have to tell you some long, stupid reason why they can't eat it. "Mexican food sets off my colitis . . ." *Who gives a shit, Peepaw?!*

Old people constantly want to give you advice that's completely worthless because their whole lives happened before the Internet. This advice often comes in the form of forty-minute anecdotes, with several sidebars about where all the people involved lived and how they individually had strokes, then died.

And yet, people think because *we're* bald, *we* are one of these decrepit dipshits. And if you insist you're thirty, not ninety, they won't believe you. Instead, they'll think you're senile and have you committed to a nursing home. Then, the first day, you'll have to beat up the oldest person you can find or you'll soon be trading sexual favors for fruit cups and Metamucil.

But while baldness makes you *look* old, you don't even have the benefits of actually *being* old, like getting fake respect for your stupid opinions, or eating dinner at 2 P.M., or being rich because everything used to be cheap back when you were young. Any elderly person who isn't wealthy from buying a house back when they cost $5 is a moron.

If I sound angry to you, believe me, you'll hate the elderly as much as I do after you've been bald ten years and laid off due to age discrimination at thirty-three because everyone thinks you're sixty-eight.

You know how I told those old people to stop reading and skip ahead? I bet those doddering stooges won't even rejoin us because they all died. Wouldn't that be hilarious?

                    *   *   *

If you're elderly and rejoining us, welcome back!

It's maddening that ten thousand fine strands of keratin placed above your forehead could be the difference between achieving your goals and failing, between living a great life and suffering a terrible one. There are many ways losing your hair impacts your day-to-day life in concrete ways, beyond emotions. And these physical effects can be equally devastating.

First, according to the BBC News, baldness causes so much stress it puts you at greater risk for heart disease than even obesity! Your bald head can literally break your heart.

Baldness also makes your senses go haywire. For a while after you go bald, like someone who loses a limb, you will feel phantom hair. You will swear it's there, swaying in the breeze. Then you'll reach back to brush it and see sparks as your fingernails shear against your dried scalp. Your eyebrows will buckle under the weight of new, unreasonable expectations and may fail you completely. In your dreams, you'll have hair—then you'll wake up bald, sweaty, and erect, which will really terrify your pets.

You will be completely betrayed by both your body and your mind. So what the hell are you supposed to do?

Undoubtedly, you're feeling all sorts of complex emojis. If you need to cry, close your windows, hug this book and do so now. If you're at your desk *at work*, that's fine too. What's the worst that can happen? Everyone already thinks you're a bizarre elderly giant baby man.

So is there any hope? Seriously, what the hell are you supposed to do?

Well, for starters, that's your last cry, baldy. Self-pity is a luxury you can no longer afford. If you have any hope of building a life, you need to face the harsh reality. Life is a zero-sum game. Everything you want, you need to take from someone with hair. There is only a finite number of good things in the world—jobs, sexual partners, Swiss cheese, infinity pools, ferrets, crèmes brûlée, Kate Uptons, electric skateboards, private jets, hallucinogenic mushrooms, dignity. Every single thing that someone with hair has is something that someone bald cannot. In the coming pages, I'll teach you to steal what's yours.

Like America before 9/11, you are in a war; you just don't realize it yet. And that war is against everyone with hair. Is that too extreme? Nope. How do I know?

I know because I lost my hair on 9/11.

2

I Went Bald on 9/11

The following is the God's-honest-truth.

It was September 10, 2001, and my life in New York City couldn't have been better. I didn't have a lot of money or a cool job or a big apartment, but I had something better: a beautiful head of long, flowing hair. I looked cool and rebellious, sort of like a male Sarah Jessica Parker. And sure, Carrie Bradshaw's New York was different from mine: she had Samantha, Charlotte, and Miranda, while I had Ruben, the half-wit living below me who would drown rats in his bathtub. But, like Carrie, I was determined to make it in the "city that doesn't sleep." I mean, I also slept a lot, but I went to futon at night with a smile, cushioned by both hope for the future and my puffy Jewfro.

On September 11, I woke up to a world I barely recognized, one that had transformed overnight from a gauzy paradise into a cruel, vicious hellscape. On my pillow I found a giant ball of hair, which had previously—every day of my life—been attached to my head. I held it in disbelief, praying it was only a dream. It wasn't.

I put on a hat and stumbled into the living room, where my room-mates sat glued to the TV for some reason. I screamed, "You won't believe what happened!" And they screamed back, "*You* won't believe what happened!" And I said, "What?" Then they said, "What?" And I said, "No, you go first," then they told me that two planes had flown into the World Trade Center, both towers had collapsed, a hijacked jet had hit the Pentagon, and another plane had crashed in Pennsylvania.

Then they asked, "But what was your thing?" And I decided I should probably save it for later.

On 9/11, there were thousands of tragedies, and devastation of such magnitude it will never be forgotten. So it sounds petty to com-plain, and yet it's true: September 11 is also the day I went bald. 9/11 was my own metaphorical 9/11, as well as being my actual 9/11, in addition to being everyone else's actual 9/11.

In the ensuing weeks and months, New Yorkers coped the only way they knew how—with candlelight vigils, and filthy tragedy sex. For men who weren't bald, the next few months were a roller coaster of sexual partners and tears. For me, however, it was a period of iso-lation as women, shaken to their core, realized that life is simply too short to fuck bald guys.

As my bald spot widened, my confidence proportionately dissi-pated. Things that seemed easy just a month earlier—work, small talk at a party, indiscriminately firing an M-16 into a chicken coop—now seemed impossible. Like some sick game of bodily whack-a-mole, the vanished hairs from my head seemed to resprout in the most inop-portune places. Nose hairs hung like vines from a trellis. I developed fur epaulets on my shoulders. My penis looked like John Oates. I believe the human body maintains the exact same number of hairs at all times. When one falls out, another grows somewhere else. You can bet the farm that Jeffrey Tambor's taint is a mess.

So when the 9/11 Commission reported that these were the scum-bags responsible for the unforgivable assault on our nation, perhaps it was only I who noticed they all had one thing in common:

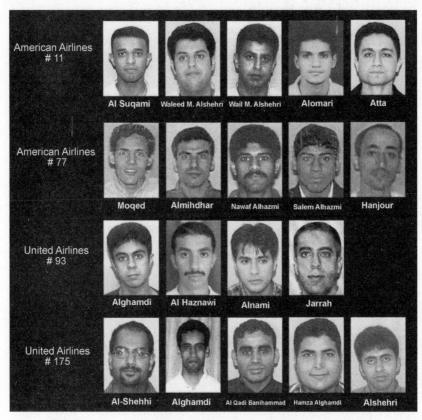

THEY **_ALL_** HAD HAIR. AND YET THE ONE PERSON THEY CAUGHT, AND
THE ONLY ONE TO BE PROSECUTED:

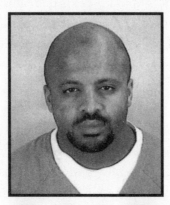

BALD.

Like America, after that day, I was never the same. The fun was gone. No amount of bombing Iraq or Afghanistan was going to bring my hair back.

As I have already told you, baldness comes from your maternal grandfather. Mine died before I was born (or I would have murdered him), but in pictures he has the self-satisfied smile of a prick who knows he's delivering misery to generations of men to come.

Grandpa Hans was a happy-go-lucky immigrant who came to this country from München with just a dollar in his pocket, and died six months later with 78 cents. But between arriving in the States and a sudden and lethal bout of tuberculosis, Hans lived life to the partialest.

At a mixer of German immigrants, he met Bertha, a young woman of low self-esteem whose parents' dream was to trade her for a mule. As is German custom, Hans and Bertha barked at one another with breath redolent of schnitzel. They had so much in common: She was fifteen years old; so was he. They both owned wool coats. They even liked the same movie, because at the time it was the only movie. One drink led to another, and soon they were doing what they call in parts of Bavaria "Das fucking."

The sexual congress was brief and unremarkable (though apparently it had made a horse witnessing it throw up, as I learned from graphic tapestries my grandmother knitted later). Hans said he'd call her, but they both knew it was a lie, since neither one of them had ever seen a phone. But what they had no way of knowing during this brief encounter was that my grandfather's baldest sperm had beat out the millions of those containing the DNA for hair.

Over one hundred years later, I walked into the velveteen lair of a Los Angeles medium, searching for closure. Maybe I could talk to Hans and learn if the afterlife had provided answers, or hair.

I'm a natural skeptic and didn't expect much from the sixty-something sorceress who definitely farted and then pretended nothing happened. "But," I asked myself, "what is the worst-case scenario? That I've just given twenty-eight thousand dollars to a fool?"

The medium turned off the light, lit some candles, and we closed our eyes. Thirty seconds later, to my surprise, the door began to rattle. I peeked and saw her twelve-year-old son asking if he could use her iPad. She whispered, "For a half hour! Not a minute longer!" then shooed him away. Then I felt a chill run over my skin. My ears pricked up. There was definitely a presence in the room. Without having given her any information, she asked, "Are you seeking a bald ghost with tuberculosis whose name begins with an H?" We had our spirit.

I told Hans I was his grandson. He asked excitedly if I owned a radio. I said I did, but it was such a small deal now that no one cared. I then quizzed Hans about his baldness. He said he was just as angry at *his* ancestors, who were just as angry at *their* ancestors. The whole thing went back so far it might have started when the earth was created two thousand years ago. I rolled my eyes, turned on the lights, and told Hans I'd see him in hell. He said, "There is no hell in the afterlife. Hell is baldness on earth."

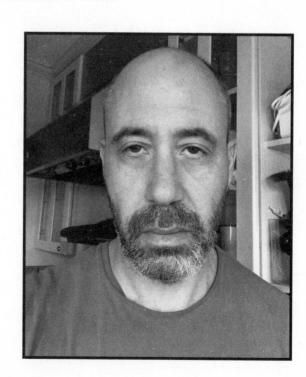

I

DIDN'T

ALWAYS

LOOK

LIKE

THIS:

I

ONCE

LOOKED

LIKE

THIS:

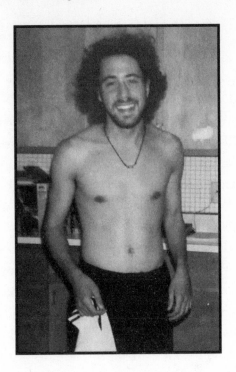

Wasn't I attractive? Well, I was seventeen, you pervert.

Look again at the younger photo. See the genuine joy? That's because I had no clue that I would someday in the not-too-distant future suffer through the Three Stages of Baldness:

1. **Anger**—this is when you realize you're going bald and you get angry.

2. **Even more anger**—this is when you look back at pictures of you from a year ago, when you thought you were really bald, only now you would kill to look like that again. And right this instant is now the most hair you'll ever have again.

3. **Even more anger**—this is when you look at the selfie from thirty seconds ago that just got you angry and you realize you just lost five more hairs.

There is no fourth stage.

No matter what life brings, you will never "get over" being bald, and that's because it makes zero sense and serves zero evolutionary purpose. Being bald makes you more prone to heat and cold and you look worse. And you're reminded of it every single time you see your own reflection. It will amplify your lows and sap the joy from your highs.

Even the birth of my first child—what should have been the most amazing moment of my life—was ruined when my daughter emerged and the doctor cooed, "Oh look, she has hair."

"Oh yeah," I wanted to scream, "because bald people aren't even human, right?!" Then she (yes, women can be doctors, you chauvinist pig) handed me my brand-new baby, and I looked into her eyes, and all I could feel was white-hot jealousy for her peach fuzz. I handed the baby right back, stormed out the door, and did a month of angry karate on the beach. To this day, all the love my children have given me pales in comparison to the envy and rage caused by their hair.

It's amazing the difference hair can make. When I had hair, job interviews ended with an offer; when I was bald, they ended with "Don't call us, we'll call you." When I had hair, bartenders gave me free drinks; when I was bald, I couldn't get served. When I had hair, Juliette Lewis once said "Hi" to me; when I was bald, Justin Long blew me off at a taqueria. But I'm sure you don't care about Julius Sharpe's troubles. You're wondering: "How will baldness affect *me*? What's *my* future going to be like?"

Real talk:

The thing you miss most when you go bald isn't combing it or brushing it or putting it in pigtails and pretending to be Dorothy from *The Wizard of Oz*. It's being visible *at all*. No one will set you up with their cute friend, invite you on a private jet, or save you from a raccoon attack. The cold, hard fact is: Nothing will ever be easy from this point onward.

You're on your own.

3

Life as a Bald Man and Why It Sucks

No one plans to be bald. It's something that's thrust upon you, like greatness or chlamydia. It's virtually impossible to prepare enough for your hair's demise. If you have anything left on top, you need to immediately throw a "hairwell party," which is basically a bachelor party for your head. Call your buddies, hit Vegas, get your hair wasted and laid, and take a bunch of pictures, because it's the last time you two are gonna see each other ever again. Your hair is dead and will only live on if an inner-city teen paints a mural of it.

The second you go bald, get ready—everyone will start assuming you're Michael Chiklis. Several times a week, people approach me on the street simply to let me know they're not impressed and don't want my autograph. Rather than bore them with an explanation of all of their misassumptions, I typically just utter Michael Chiklis's catchphrase, "Hi, I'm Michael Chiklis."

Some things you learn immediately. For instance, baldness makes you look enraged and everyone assumes you're angry all the time. They'll ask, "You doing okay?" Never ask a bald man how he's doing. He's doing bad. He's bald. Move on.

Other things take time to learn. Like: Never wave back at anyone. They're definitely waving at the person behind you. No one's saying "Hi" to you; you're bald.

On top of looking like a Ban roll-on deodorant, there are other small joys you won't notice you're missing until much later. You can't whip your hair back and forth when you blast Willow Smith. You can't drop the top of a convertible and feel the breeze through your 'do. You'll never be pulled onstage at a Beyoncé concert. No one will ever brush your bangs out of your eyes and kiss you on a pile of seaweed at a public beach. You can't meld your hair into dreadlocks with another person, creating a pseudo-Jamaican Siamese twin.

No more college professors will see you as a potential seduction target in return for a C+ after you completely failed the midterm. No one will bring you Gatorade when you barf. Don't bother hitchhiking—no one will stop. There will be no nationwide manhunt when you go missing. (The best you can hope for is Xeroxed posters, tops.) No one with a cool house will ever ask you to housesit. Dogs will bite you. You'll never be offered weed. Lifeguards will let you drown because they think you're a buoy.

Then, there are the larger consequences. Bald men almost never sign giant, exclusive modeling contracts; we're the last picked at orgies; and in rock bands, we're forced to be the drummer. Every time we play charades, people think the clue is "A bald asshole." We are charged the same airline baggage fees, even though we're not packing any shampoos or mousses. I can't even tell you how many times people have said, "Get off our ski slope, you bald Jew!" (I suspect something else may be at play here.)

You no longer get to go to a barber, which hurts on two fronts. First, you miss the camaraderie. I don't know about you, but every time I sit down in that barber's chair, I instantly tell him everything that's been going on with me sexually since the last trim. It's a chance to brag about being awesome to a guy who's pretending to be enthusiastic because you're paying him.

And if you're as emotionally repressed as I am, your barber may be the only other male to touch you your entire life. Your spirit craves that contact, that hairy reassuring hand on your shoulder that says, "A real man, the kind of man who eats beef stew and has no idea who or what One Direction is, cares about you."

Plus, without hair, what the hell are you supposed to do in the shower? A bald man in the shower has no agenda. He is a ronin, a scalp samurai with no master. You're standing there, a naked doofus, surrounded by shampoos you can't use, under a tiny fake rainstorm. What, are you going to take a *bath*? You're really gonna steep yourself in a tea brewed from your own filth? That's disgusting.

However, baldness does open up new opportunities to be creative in previously mundane situations. And with a little bit of thought, there is *plenty* you can do in a shower. Rather than obsess over what's missing, I like to focus on what I have and really detail my genitals. It's easy, free, and you can do it too. Here's how:

1. **Rid your undercarriage of dust, dirt, and debris.** An old toothbrush, a foaming agent, and a little elbow grease will help restore your penis to its original color.

2. **Condition the ball skin as you would leather and vinyl.** After all, we humans are basically leather. You want your testicles to be so smooth and supple that a 1950s dad would sit in them like an armchair, get annihilated on martinis, and read the paper while his terrified family hides in the kitchen, praying he's not displeased.

3. **Apply a sealant.** A few thin coats of shellac will help preserve your reconditioned taint and bring your peener and nutsack to a high shine.

4. **Buff and polish to perfection.** I think you understand what I'm telling you to do: masturbate.

While you may feel desperate and completely out of control over what others say is "just hair," this agony is *not* irrational and makes complete sense when viewed through the prism of "loss aversion." "Loss aversion" is a theory based on the work of psychologists Daniel Kahneman (bald) and Amos Tversky (hair) for which they won a Nobel Prize, which is kind of like a Country Music Award but for thinking.

"Loss aversion" says that the agony of losing something is far greater than the pleasure of gaining it. People hate losing far more than they enjoy winning. The real-world implications are simple. The hurt of losing a hundred dollars at blackjack is greater than the pleasure of winning a hundred dollars. The agony of losing your keys supersedes the joy of finding them. Crashing an airplane still feels bad, even if you've landed a bunch of them safely.

You, the bald man, are experiencing loss every single day, watching your precious hair go down the drain. My theory, for which I'm hoping to win at least a People's Choice, is that the agony of losing your hair outweighs whatever joy you can get in other areas of your life. Success doesn't feel like success when you're still bald after. No triumph is so big you wouldn't immediately trade it for hair.

Personally, baldness destroyed my stand-up comedy career and I had to become a writer. And while I'm able to make a living, it's a tempered joy. To me, it proves people are okay with what I have to say, they just don't want to look at me while I say it.

The discrepancy between who baldness makes you and who you could be with hair is a form of discrimination. But if you, a bald man, complain about being discriminated against, you'll be told you're not a real minority and maybe even fired for insensitivity. Try getting laid then! (Actually, that's not a bad time to try getting laid because you're already being fired. What are they gonna do, take away a job you don't have?)

Discrimination is everywhere, beginning in the Bible. Samson becomes weak after cutting his hair, for example. In Kings II 2:23, as Elisha goes to Bethel, some boys jeer him—they sayeth, "Get ye out of here, baldy!" In U.S. history, there have only been five bald presidents out of forty-five, and one was John Quincy Adams, who was basically a shittier version of John Adams and shouldn't even count. And, in movies and TV, almost every villain is bald, including Gollum, Bane, Voldemort, Lex Luthor, Sméagol, Walter White, Mr. Burns, Dr. Evil, Tony Soprano, Thanos, and Dr. Phil.

TV shows and movies imply these men are bald because they're evil, but they have it entirely backward. They're evil because they're bald! The insecurity and rage of baldness stoked by an uncaring and scornful society is what turned them against everyone. As noted in *Baldness: A Social History*, study after study shows men are negatively perceived because they're bald. These characters aren't intrinsically evil. Like all human beings, they start out good. It's only once they begin going bald and they're treated differently that they want to destroy the world.

There exists no greater example of "hair bias" than the movie *Apocalypse Now*. In the film, Marlon Brando plays Colonel Kurtz, a bald man having a fun time in the Cambodian jungle during the Vietnam War. Of course, the U.S. government can't tolerate bald joy and sends a ragtag group of trigger-happy soldiers with hair (Martin Sheen, Laurence Fishburne, and a bunch of nobodies) to restore Kurtz to his rightful place at the bottom of the hair-erarchy.

The group finally reaches Kurtz and what they find horrifies them: A bald man has built a lovely compound where people worship him and make nice dinners. The ultimate sign of a world gone insane is bald happiness. If Kurtz had hair, undoubtedly the troops would have said, "Hey, cool house!", been on their way, and sent a thank-you note a week later on fancy stationery. Instead, they murder Kurtz, then leave without even making their beds.

To me, "The horror, the horror" is perhaps the way we demonize bald men with Asian wives.

The film is widely misinterpreted as an allegory about the U.S. government's involvement in the Vietnam War. However, more recent work by hairless film scholars has reached an entirely different conclusion: *Apocalypse Now* is Stanley Kubrick's three-hour-long tacit confession of the hunting and killing of bald men for sport, a sick secret practice in Hollywood since the age of the talkies. Fueled by whiskey, ether, and a love of eugenics, and covered up by the major studios, bald hunting began when Jimmy Stewart, Lana Turner, and Errol Flynn used to drive their matching Opel Olympias down Hollywood Boulevard, and whoever ran over the most bald men "won" and would get free unlimited malteds at the Chasen's soda counter. The bodies would be tossed into crude shallow graves on Hollywood Boulevard, which back then was mostly farmland, as it remains today.

Ever notice during the Academy Awards that the Oscar statue is bald? This began as an inside joke. The trophies weren't awarded based on the films at all—they were given to the actors, directors, and producers who'd run over the most bald guys, who they'd derisively refer to as "Oscars" because of O-shaped scars (O-scars) left by tire treads on their chests.

But it's not just the Academy that's antibald—it's all of pop culture. Think about who we call "Superman." Every hairless man should hate Superman's guts. Why is everyone so against Lex Luthor and so gaga for Superman? First of all, Superman is a fucking alien from outer space. That's who you want in power? All we really know about him is his parents took one look at him and bailed. But everyone's ready to put him in charge over a guy who's actually *from earth* just because that guy is bald and Superman has hair! Metropolis First! Make Metropolis Great Again!

Superman already has good looks, a girlfriend, and a job as a reporter, but that's not enough for him. No, it just gets in Superman's craw that a powerful bald man has big ambitions while Superman works at a dumb newspaper that's probably going to be taken over by Buzzfeed any second. Sure, Lex Luthor wants world domination—because he's really smart and deserves it! He's not like Superman, born with superpowers! Everything Lex Luthor has, he earned! Superman is basically a cultural imperialist from Krypton, but everyone favors him over Lex Luthor because "bald" equals "evil."

And now, I have a confession to make: Baldness has made *me* kinda evil.

Only once you lose it do you realize most of the affection, compassion, and companionship in your life is granted to you because of your hair. And learning that love is conditional rattles your worldview to the core.

Going bald annihilated my moral compass. Before balding, I'd feel sorry for a homeless person and maybe give him a dollar and whatever cheese I had on me. Now, though, if a bum has hair, I find myself screaming, "You lethargic hobo! If I had your lustrous coiffure, I'd be a trillionaire!" This has led to knife fight after knife fight.

Then there are the victims of tornadoes. My compassion for them is determined not by their plight, but by their hairline—your house blew away? Must be nice. My hair blew away. At least your thing was insured. I see an innocent person with great hair who got duped by a Ponzi scheme and think, "Ha-ha, Kevin Bacon, I'm glad Bernie Madoff took your money." I don't believe anyone with hair has any right to their problems. Also, I feel like if I could somehow reacquire *my* hair, all my social and financial problems would go away.

I was a happy-go-lucky kid. I didn't want everyone else to die until I was twenty-nine and it was clear even the hair on my own head wanted to jump ship. At that point, why wouldn't I want everyone to suffer as much as I did? Now, I love nothing better than when a person with hair returns from a Hawaiian vacation where it rained the whole time or a guy with a ponytail has his nose ripped off by a chimpanzee. (I privately suspect many of these face-ripping "chimpanzees" are actually just bald guys with bad posture.)

But I don't think this evil is intrinsic to me. I think it was learned, because over and over again, the media hammers home the "evil" of baldness. Under his helmet, Darth Vader was bald, so we're supposed to celebrate when the Death Star is blown up, but what the hell? A lot of people worked really hard to build that thing. How would you feel if you installed the windows on the Death Star and they all exploded? Especially when you bought that expensive truck that had those extra glass-carrying scaffolds on each side? Now maybe you understand why *Star Wars* is stupid.

The most maddening aspect of baldness is that all your crazed paranoia turns out to be true, which only fuels more crazed paranoia. I call this "hairanoia." In a survey by the *Journal of American Medical Association Facial Plastic Surgery* (great magazine—the centerfold is always a bashed-in face) comparing bald people to those with hair, haired people rated higher in perception of attractiveness, successfulness, and approachability.

These benefits amount to a sort of "hair privilege." What is hair privilege? It's the unearned benefits those with hair get over bald people as we all travel through our daily lives. Smiles, doors held open, extra pancakes at Denny's, free shampoo and conditioner at hotels, and to bring it back to topic, nonevil roles in movies. The portrayal of bald as evil creates a circular effect. Bald people *become* evil because the media shows them that's how they *should* behave. Our jails are full of bald "criminals" who, I believe, would never have strayed from the right side of the law if they had hair. Every bald prisoner should immediately be given a million dollars, a blanket, and a gallon of orange juice and set free.

If you're not bald, it's important to realize you see the world from the perspective of "hair privilege" and you need to check this immediately. If you're white and talking to a bald black guy, you're also seeing things from "white privilege" and you need to check your "hairy white privilege." If you're Asian, I honestly have no clue what you should do.

People will attempt to "hairsplain" to you, "Oh, it's no big deal. I don't even notice you're bald," as though *their* (or if you're from

Arkansas, *there*) experience of *your* (Arkansas, *you're*) baldness is more important than your own. Of course they don't notice you're bald, any more than you or I notice which ants are having a bad day! Those with hair exist so far above us, they don't see us scurrying around below. The person who is actually experiencing the baldness is trapped inside the bald head, unable to get out.

Losing hair privilege results in fewer jobs, fewer dates, and way fewer "likes" on Instagram. The only people who "like" our photos are other desperate bald guys with the tacit understanding of "Now you like *my* photo." So now we're engaged in an endless "like" jerkoff fest with a bunch of bald garbage (no offense) with zero payoff.

It's harder for bald people to mate, climb the corporate ladder, and almost impossible to get out of a traffic violation by showing your tits. There's a musical *Hair;* there's no musical *Bald*. Bald actors can't even land roles playing evil bald people! These parts are stolen by actors with hair who shave their heads in a crude caricature of a hairless pate. Walter White of *Breaking Bad* is one of the great "baldface" performances of all time. An actor with hair, Bryan Cranston, plays a bald man in a kind of bald minstrel show. Yet this "hairwashing" barely makes a ripple in Hollywood, where they seem to have their heads up their asses trying to convince us Jon Hamm is funny. Just let him be serious. Hamm'll be fine!

Why didn't Walter White, the Emmy-winning role of a lifetime, go to Ron Howard, Billy Zane, or Jason Alexander? The ugly truth is: Because they've been "baldlisted."

And whether you know it or not, so have you. You've been passed over, fired, or never even considered because you're bald. Bald guys sometimes even make less than women! You can't even benefit from thousands of years of sexism! How unfair is that? And yet, sit down next to any woman and say, "I know how you feel, sister," and it's amazing how quickly she grabs her bag and summons a security guard, who's also usually bald but will beat you anyway to prove to his hairy overlords he's not some bald sympathizer.

So yes, it's not all in your head (and none of it's *on* your head). Baldness hurts your chances of success in life. Tough talk? Sure. But better you know it and believe it than buy people's lies about how they didn't even notice you're bald.

So what's the solution?

Therapy? Don't throw your money away. Paying some person with a giant amount of grad school debt to pretend to be your friend will never work because at the end of every session, time's up and you're still bald. And having a bald therapist is even worse. You list everything that's wrong with you and the entire time he's agreeing, "I know, I know," then you both leave depressed.

So if therapy is off the agenda, how about pure anger? Yes, your anger can be harnessed to destroy others and make everyone else feel worse than you, and that certainly helps. But, while other people's suffering is always great, it isn't quite the same thing as your own actual happiness.

So where to begin? I know you're scared, lost, and confused, but nothing good will ever happen for you if you stay locked up in your room, refreshing baldness message boards. You need to get out there and compete against all those giant hairholes and take what's yours.

But how can you possibly overcome the extreme bias we face? How will you ever be seen as anything other than an albino dildo? The first step is: You need to get a personality, and fast!!

Handy List of Things That Are Worse than Being Bald

- Swimming through stingray cum

- The Civil War

- Almost getting a spare in bowling

- When three or more people want to split the check

- YouTube celebrities

- When a plumber or mechanic can tell you have no idea what he's talking about

- Accidentally eating used kitty litter

- Overcooked final meal on death row

- Any wedding ceremony that takes longer than three minutes

- Getting a Frisbee stuck on a roof, then trying to knock it off with one of your shoes, then also getting your shoe stuck on the roof

- Someone telling you a video is funny, then watching you as you watch it

- Wet croutons

- Pillows with knit wisdom on them

- Lambskin condoms

- When you can't tell if you're still on hold so you say, "Hello?" and the other person says, "I'm still here," and now they know you're a coward who can't be alone

- A person with a clipboard in front of the supermarket

- Ebola

4

How to Get a Personality, and Fast!

Look in a mirror. Go on, look. Pick out your nicest feature. Maybe you have deep blue eyes. Maybe you got them kissin' lips. Maybe you possess totally sweet, hairless nose holes. Really focus on that thing that makes you special and appreciate your own intrinsic beauty. Now fill your heart with love, and ask yourself, "When people look at me, what do they see?"

The answer is: They see a bald fuck.

They don't care about any "features" you have besides your dumb bald head. That'd be like expecting someone to notice the mint-condition door handles on the burning carcass of a Pontiac that just exploded on the freeway. Your bald head is that smoldering rubble. Anyone looking at you is just rubbernecking. The second people see you, their brain sends a message: "Bald guy, unfuckable."

So if you want to have a happy life, friends, and sex one more time before death, you are going to have to change that message by getting yourself a personality.

"I'm me. Isn't that enough?"

Nope! On top of competing with everyone with hair, you are going to need to stand out from the world's 750 million bald guys, and *they all look exactly like you!* Exactly! Sometimes I'm at a party and I think another bald guy *is* me, and he gets very confused when I'm hungry and I stuff a dumpling in his mouth. And I'm wondering, "Why am I still hungry if I just saw myself eat a dumpling?" If *we* can't tell us apart, how do we expect eligible women to do so?

Plus, you're not just up against bald guys and men with hair, you're also competing against women *for* women! Bisexuality is way ahead of bald guys on most lady's lists and rightfully so. And of course these women are way better at sex with women than we are, because they get to practice on themselves. Lesbianism is basically insider trading!

Most women with self-respect won't sleep with a bald man. But for those who will, they have their pick of the entire 750 million, so it's very important you be the number-one bald guy out there. I call it "being the best of the worst."

Your only hope to stand out in a positive way—apart from appearance—is a personality.

Most people think "a personality" is some sort of intrinsic thing. But on the contrary, a personality is a series of tricks you use so people don't judge you by your looks.

Cavemen all looked the same—hairy, filthy, and covered with years' worth of their own dried shit—and consequently everyone *was* the same. This had some advantages—no one could ever tell who farted—and some disadvantages—no one knew who anyone was, so when you did something spectacular, everyone thought Og did it, even though he's a fucking moron. Evolution dictated we develop personalities so we could tell ourselves from others, and so we could tell others apart from other others.

Your very survival is at stake. Cellphones pose an existential threat to the bald man. There has never been a worse time to be bald. Two hundred years ago, it wasn't that big a deal. People only met like twenty other people their entire lives, then died at twenty-six, so they were bald for maybe a year, tops. Pictures weren't even a thing. If you were lucky, you got oil-painted maybe twice in your life. If you slipped the artist a nickel, he'd add hair. And as bald as you were, you can bet it was probably better than what was going on with everyone else. Who's going to judge your baldness when they have scurvy, ringworms, and a face full of mumps?

Now, unfortunately, most of the diseases that made everyone else look like shit—smallpox, bubonic plague, cholera—have been eradicated in spite of the hard work of Jenny McCarthy. But baldness persists. And we live in a time when everyone, even total nobodies, is photographed more than ever. These pictures are spread everywhere across social media and viewed billions of times a day by people who are supposed to be working. Fifteen years ago, if you'd taken a picture of yourself, people would have called you an egomaniac and beaten you with your own camera. Now, selfies are the currency of our time.

In order to prevent bald men from going extinct in an appearance-obsessed technocracy, we will need to adapt and evolve, with traits that distract from our hairlessness. A personality makes baldness the *second* thing people notice about you (or preferably the hundredth, but let's not aim too high).

This strategy is illustrated at its simplest by Mikhail Gorbachev having a giant fake birthmark on his head. He's no longer "the bald guy," he's "the birthmark guy," which is, if anything, worse. But it demonstrates that something prominent in the middle of your forehead can point people's attention away from your baldness.

Likewise, you're going to need something notable about you so the first thing that comes to mind when people see you isn't "bald." You could be, "Bill, the air guitar champion who always wears a graduation gown," or "Don, who swallows baked potatoes whole," or "Kent, the guy with the giant spacer earrings who was attacked by his own Gila monster."

You can survive and even thrive in this age, and not just because those two things rhyme. You will simply make sure that your looks, which completely suck, are eclipsed by your personality, which we'll make sure doesn't suck as much.

Personalities have three components. They are:

1. What you do

2. What you say

3. How you look

That's it. These three things are all that separate us from doorknobs. Let's investigate them now.

5

What People with Personalities Do

Once you're bald, it's almost impossible to get attention.

HEY! I SAID, "ONCE YOU'RE BALD, IT'S ALMOST IMPOSSIBLE TO GET ATTENTION!" See? Even I can barely get it now.

This is why you see so many bald men in the know on unicycles, hang gliders, Segways, and every other stupid mode of transportation. It's why you'll find baldies playing the accordion, organizing "Big Lebowski" festivals, strolling with Great Danes, or participating in adult kickball leagues. It's why Joe Rogan and Dana White won't shut up about MMA. You have to make people notice you for any reason other than being bald.

To gain attention, you're going to need to quirk it up like you never have before. There's an easy way to come up with ideas: Walk around for a day and make a mental note of all the people you find annoying. Likely you'll see people riding electric scooters, doing Tai Chi, roller-skating with pythons around their necks, and bobbing their head way too hard in drum circles . . . basically anyone doing anything that makes them seem so happy it pisses you off. It doesn't matter that they have your attention because they're annoying; all that matters is that they have your attention. So copy them.

If you're lost because there are too many choices, I'll solve it for you right now. A miniature horse costs $500. Look at this fucking thing:

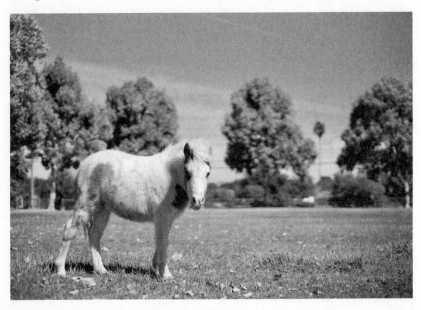

You're telling me if you walk around with this cute-as-shit motherfucker, no woman is going to talk to you? They will all talk to you because they want to touch this tiny goddamn horse. Your bald head will fade into the background the second they see this little stud munching hay. Anything smaller than a regular thing is inherently interesting. Kittens, mini cupcakes, baby shoes . . . It's why people are so into chihuahuas and Bruno Mars.

You ever hear someone say, "I'm so sick of these tiny horses!"? Hell no. So set up shop in a public place with your equine dwarf and start brushing the wee guy's tail. Pretty soon you'll be surrounded by babes and kids. Tell the kids to go screw and let the babes stay.

If this catches on, and you find that the world is overrun with bald men leading tiny horses around by their bridles, downsize to a micro pig. Once there's too many micro pigs, get a pygmy goat. Keep going smaller and end when you buy a half-size amoeba.

Or maybe it's easier to get attention with a big, friendly dog? Good thinking. There are many different breeds of dog, but you'll want a golden retriever, because they all look exactly the same. You'll also want to buy six at once, keep them in six different apartments all over the city, and give them all the same name. You'll see why this is important in a minute.

Once you have your golden(s), you'll start to see the same people walking their dogs every day. As you make small talk with them, your dogs will sniff each other's butts and start humping, because they don't share our stupid hang-ups. After this happens enough times, the two owners will eventually have sex just because they feel stupid their dogs are having more sex than they are. With six dogs in six separate locations, you'll have six sex situations going and can narrow it down to the best two or three.

One problem, though: Dogs die. And guess what happens next? The woman who's sleeping with you because her dog is sleeping with your dog will leave you for a guy with a nice, alive dog. Fortunately, you're prepared, because you have six identical dogs with the same name. When the dog she *thinks* is your dog is run over by a car or gets a weird cancer, simply rotate in one of the replacements and sell the apartment where that dog was living. If this sounds like too much work and responsibility for you, then you're not mature enough to have sex anyway.

In that case, here are a few other great identity-creating activities to try out.

Square Dancing

Square dances are ideal for bald men, because anyone who shows up to one is clearly a gambling addict who's hit rock bottom. Since people aren't allowed to pick partners, they will be forced to pair up with you. As the only male participant with teeth, you will have your pick of octogenarian widows. Also, everyone is wearing giant cowboy hats, so no one will know you're bald until after, when you're all getting into your pickup trucks to drunk-drive home.

Wine Tasting

This is where you sample twenty liquids that taste exactly the same but try to point out minuscule differences to prove you are some kind of genius at sipping things. People will pretend they taste "hints" of this and "notes" of that. "I detect hints of limestone, tennis ball, rattlesnake, and maybe notes of old bathrobe? This would pair well with me falling down the stairs and no one finding me for two weeks because I live alone."

Here's what all wines taste like: grapes. Every single wine in the history of wines is made from one ingredient: grapes, and that's what grapes taste like: grapes. But saying that would mean you're not sophisticated, you're just a bunch of drunks listing nouns, so instead claim you taste nectarine and fresh-cut grass and no one will bat an eyelash. After three glasses, you'll meet tons of people who say their marriage didn't work out because their spouse stopped listening to them when, in reality, it failed because their spouse *started* listening to them. Then you'll all get in your Priuses to drunk-drive home.

Hot Air Ballooning

Imagine taking a date up in a hot air balloon. How cool would that be? Just you, her, subzero temperatures, a wicker basket, and a giant torch.

There are FAA requirements to get a hot air balloon license, but honestly, you think there are hot air balloon cops riding around in cop balloons up there who are going to stop you? Some sheriff in another balloon's gonna be like, "Pull over that balloon!"? Where would you even pull over—a cloud? You'll be fine.

Cycling

You've probably noticed a bunch of people riding around your town, clad in spandex, who have somehow convinced themselves that even though they're all middle-aged and chubby, they're professional bike racers. This is a good tribe for you to join. You'll get out in the sunshine, get some exercise, and meet people whose prostate horror stories will make baldness seem like the work of an angel.

There's more: Given the high rate of bicyclists being hit by cars, any woman who runs you over will likely feel so guilty afterward that she'll *have* to date you for a month. Back when I was single, I would crash through every windshield I could. This would invariably lead to an exchange of information and, voilà! I had a woman's number! And you won't need to go through the whole "Hi, you probably don't remember me . . ." spiel. You destroyed her Jetta! She's definitely gonna remember you!

But taking up these "hobbies" won't be quite enough—you'll also need to say some stuff, or else people will naturally assume you're a mute who was abandoned by a bankrupt circus with a tiny horse next to a hot air balloon.

Before we get to what to say, I just want to point out that there is a way to have it all: parrots. Parrots have beautiful plumage, and they can memorize over 1,500 words. The average English conversation uses just 1,000 words. That means you can teach your parrot to talk, plus 500 extra medical terms so he can be your literal wingman as you try to hook up with a female doctor. Let those two blab away about bladder cystectomies while you sit there fantasizing you're an NBA player, which is basically all any of us really wants.

The only potential pitfall is the woman and parrot, sharing a deep love of medicine, will realize they no longer need you as a middleman. Then she takes your parrot. You can sue her, but it's their word against yours in court, and when the parrot takes the stand, he's definitely lying under oath because swearing on the Bible means nothing to him. You forgot to teach him the word "God."

6

What to Say

If possible, never say anything. Most people's definition of a great conversation is when they said tons of stuff and the other person listened. Listening is simply not talking, then saying "Uh- huh" every few seconds. These uh-huhs will reassure the speaker that you're not dead, so they can keep going. People get in trouble all the time for talking, but no one's ever gotten yelled at or fired for listening too much.

However, sometimes you will be compelled to talk because the other person will stop yammering away in order to eat, or have an asthma attack. You must never allow any silence in any conversation, because your date will interpret this as a sign you don't have enough in common. They'll delete you from their phone, so when you text them a few days later, they'll text back, "Who dis?" Then you'll text them, "Dis Jeff," and they'll never reply. Then you'll have to spend the rest of your life wondering whether they didn't want to talk to you or they were raptured after "Dis Jeff."

Anyway, when it's your turn to speak, the strategy is simple. All anyone wants to hear is compliments.

Quick exercise: I want you to list five nonhair-related compliments you wish someone would give to you:

_____

_____

_____

_____

_____

Great. Now memorize them and constantly say them to other people. Don't worry if they're true or not. They probably won't be. Most people stink. But if you can say them without violently twitching, people will *think* they're true, and people who are thinking about how great *they* are aren't thinking about how bald *you* are.

However, if, after knowing someone a few years, they start to realize you're reusing the same five compliments, you'll need to find new areas of conversation. It's important to be aware there are many things you *can't* talk about.

The following topics are absolutely no-go: religion, politics, money, babies, family, current events, gender, sexuality, ethnicity, books, drugs, music, peanut allergies, adult diapers, Darwinism, Marxism, sadism, classicism, feminism, racism, guns, climate change, corporal punishment, capital punishment, Daylight Savings Time, blogs, celebrities, Trump, Obama, Hillary, the electoral college, abortion, Israel, Palestine, culture, sports, nutrition, alternative medicine, cars, history, art, Facebook, Instagram, Twitter, assisted suicide, immigration, the national anthem, the regional anthem, any local anthems, the gold standard, welfare, prostitution, bridge trolls, bog monsters, Sasquatch, ghosts, animal rights, vegetable wrongs, affirmative action, free trade, net neutrality, NAFTA, waterboarding, drones, the zodiac, grammar, cereal, Gwyneth Paltrow, hair, gluten, movies, she-devils, Pap smears, spontaneous combustion, Elon Musk, and, finally, anything related to any aspect of her or you.

All any of these subjects could possibly do is alienate, terrify, or enrage. If you had hair, maybe you could pull it off, but since you're bald, you'd be excoriated and your name would become an angry hashtag on Twitter. Better to be #BaldQuiet.

So what to do if these topics come up? Simple: Smile, shake your head, and say, "It's crazy." That's it. You're just an average, simple bald guy, bemused at the folly of humankind.

So what can you talk about?

There are only two topics of conversation available to a bald man:

1. Restaurants

2. Places you want to travel

As a married guy, trust me, that's enough to fill a lifetime of talk. Ninety percent of being in a relationship is deciding what to have for dinner and the other 10 percent is thinking of countries you want to see but will never get to. Every night, she'll ask what you're in the mood for. Here's what you're in the mood for: whatever she's in the mood for. You should always say everything "sounds yummy!" no matter how weird it feels to yell "yummy!" Be permanently positive. Spend all your time reading online reviews of restaurants, then quote the best things as if you thought of them. That's personality.

The good news is that all restaurants are basically the same— they have roast chicken and serve Brussels sprouts with bacon. The special is usually sea bass, and it's awful. The waiter will always blink too much and half the stuff you order will be completely botched.

Thousands of people have licked the silverware, and that's revolting. Despite these flaws, always be positive. "I hear that place is good" is one thing to say. Another is "Oh man, I can't wait to try that place." If she says the food's not good, you say you didn't notice because it's so nice being with her, you little charmer.

Before you dig into that roast chicken, though, here's the most important thing: *You cannot gain one fucking ounce.* You can't be both fat and bald. Your ideal look is "Guy who was shipwrecked six years ago."

This isn't a diet book, so all I'll say is, I've tried everything—wheat-free, Atkins, Weight Watchers, vegan, even Bethenny Frankel's exclusive "seagull and olive diet" (eat as many seagulls as you want, plus eight olives a day)—but only one thing has ever worked, which is: *Don't eat anything.*

Given that you're on a date and not eating, your date will likely say, "Try some." That's when you lie: "I've already had so much, you have the rest." On top of *you* staying thin, *she'll* start to put on weight, her self-esteem will go down, then she'll feel like she's out of options and has to stay with you. It's the ultimate win-win!

Which brings us to exercise. Here's one area where baldness works in your favor. The constant hammering anxiety that baldness engenders raises your heart rate, jacks up your adrenaline, and pins your endocrine system into overdrive, mimicking the effects of sprinting. Your fears are a CrossFit gym you carry everywhere, all the time!

7

How to Look

What makes a tree a Christmas tree? We hold no special sentiment for the tree itself (on the contrary, we murder it to put it in our home). It's the decoration that elevates it from dead plant to object of affection. How could you likewise be something people would proudly display in their living room? By getting a box of stuff out of the attic and decorating your head.

Think of yourself as Mr. Potato Head. He has a vast array of glasses, hats, eyes, ears, and noses. Why? Because he's bald! But by constantly changing his looks, he's able to compete for children's attention versus iPads even though he's just a fake potato.

You are essentially a giant fake potato of a human being. Your head is your palate, and you are Picasso (who was bald, so his portraits of other people were basically "Fuck you, this is what I think *you* look like!"), so don't be afraid to pierce it, paint it, throw stuff on top of it, try beards, sideburns, whatever. You're already at rock bottom, you might as well throw some ziti at the wall and see what sticks. Get that nose ring! Tattoo your eyeballs and make your mother cry! Grow a scraggly beard, wear a sleeveless shirt, and say you're a *Duck Dynasty* guy! Cut off your ears, intentionally contract rabies, and attack everyone at a Waffle House! The possibilities are endless!

Where to start? Perhaps with the two easiest tried-and-tested ways bald men can distract attention from the tops of their heads: fauxhawks and hats.

Fauxhawks

This maneuver only works if you still have some hair left on top. If you do, the fauxhawk can help you eke out two more years while you scramble to get your affairs in order before completely balding. It's a hip, modern take on the combover for Millennials and Generation Z.

There are three main problems with the old-school combover. Number one, it looks stupid. And number two, you can't jump into a pool, which is the only classy way to fart at a resort. Three is that employing the combover is like trying to cover up nuclear waste with a sign that says NO NUCLEAR WASTE. People weren't even *thinking* about nuclear waste until they saw the sign, but now that's all they'll see. Same with a combover—it's the nuclear waste sign of bald deception. Because it draws attention to a disaster, it's a solution that's worse than the problem.

Where my revolutionary fauxhawk technique differs from the combover is in the intricacy of the deception. One combover is bad; what nobody ever expects is *two* combovers. Or three combovers! That's exactly what the fauxhawk is. The brazen nature of the crime is so staggering it defies perception and goes unseen: three combovers, swirled together in the middle of your head, creating a mound that is solidified with gel. It's a frigging armed robbery with a tank in broad daylight.

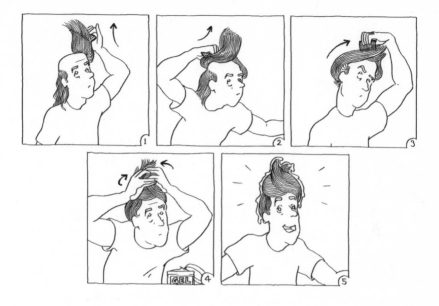

Just as a cubic zirconia is indistinguishable from a real diamond except by a gemologist, this man-made hair Kilimanjaro can't be told from the real thing except by the discerning critical eye of another fauxhawked bald man.

But here's where you learn the bald have a few unwritten rules. When two bald men enter an intersection, the balder one has right of way. During a disaster, those with more hair—and thus more reason to live—take precedence over the completely glabrous. And most important, while bald men don't have unity or friendship, we have something perhaps more effective: fear-based détente. We don't blow up each other's (bald) spots. No bald man will ever point out your fauxhawk, lest you unmask his fauxhawk and both your lives are obliterated. So enjoy your fauxhawk while it lasts, which unfortunately won't be long.

As autumn follows summer and leaves turn brown, wither, and die, so too will your fauxhawk droop, thin, then fall to the ground in a pile that your dad will give you $20 to rake into a trash bag. At this point, there's only one option left.

Hats

How convenient that it's socially acceptable to wear giant things on our heads! Hats date back to 3200 B.C., when it occurred to the first bald ancient Egyptians to build tiny stone pyramids to cover their exposed craniums. These early balds were glad for the shelter and others were grateful they didn't have to look at them. The pharaoh himself decreed it "a total win-win." So-called "hats" quickly caught on and became such a craze that many scholars believe the Great Sphinx of Giza was actually a Lids.

Hats were largely forgotten during the Dark Ages as people became so stupid they no longer even knew how to use their arms to put things on top of their heads. In the Middle Ages, hats made a resurgence as a way to convey social status. You either wore a crown (king) or a bale of hay and cholera feces on your head (peasant). Hats then took on a military application, so soldiers knew they were killing the right people on the battlefield. The phrase "Shoot the guys in red hats" reduced arrow friendly-fire deaths by over 99.99999 percent.

Soldiers who returned from battle wore their hats to let women know they'd been in the war, which was the first known use of hats as fashion. From there hats exploded: The tricorn hat, the derby, the straw boater—it seems as though a new hat came out every fifty years or so, almost too fast for society to keep up. There are now almost ten kinds to choose from. Each hat broadcasts a message about the wearer that subliminally communicates your whole backstory.

The Cowboy Hat, or Stetson

Wearing a cowboy hat means you don't have to shoehorn "Just so you know, I'm a cowboy" into every conversation. The Stetson is enough to convey you're a salt-of-the-earth real man who does manual labor and is secretly gay when he goes to the mountains.

Remember when Anna Nicole Smith was alive and one of the most beautiful women in the world? Then she married an eighty-eight-year-old oilman? That's the power of the cowboy hat. Women know anyone wearing it might have struck oil and become a billionaire, so they'll at least have to marry you and wait 'til you die to find out.

The Surgical Cap

Want people to think you're a successful professional who saves lives and helps their fellow man? Swipe some surgical caps next time you're at the doctor's office. Don't worry if you're on an airplane and a stewardess screams, "Is anyone a doctor? This man is having a heart attack!" Just raise your hand and try to help. If you succeed, great. If not, real doctors lose patients all the time. It's no big deal. Just do what they do in a real hospital: "Nurse, please inform the family while I sneak out back to my Jaguar."

The Captain's Hat

Would you like people to think you make pornography, or recorded "Muskrat Love" with Tennille? Captain's hat all the way.

The Beanie

Tell people you're a professional DJ when really you're an Uber driver with a three-star rating.

The Baseball Cap

The baseball cap is a miraculous accelerator of social relationships. Wearing the same cap as a sports team instantly joins you to a tribe of people who will hug, high-five, and even blow you when your team wins. There are hundreds of teams to choose from, but here are what I believe to be the three best for beginners.

New York Yankees

Don't know much about sports? Don't worry, neither do most Yankees fans. They almost all come from somewhere stupid and either hate their hometown or are ashamed of it, so they wear this cap to be associated with a long tradition of winning they had nothing to do with. A Yankees hat conveniently provides an opportunity to network with almost anyone from stockbrokers to the homeless and ensures you'll get punched less whenever you're in New York (except Queens).

Cleveland Browns

Being bald may make you feel like a loser, but you're always a winner next to Cleveland Browns fans. The Browns are less a team and more a group of guys who can't play football all wearing the same shirt. They've sucked for decades. Their most famous play in the last fifty years is a fumble. The hat reminds people, "A bald guy can't be the worst thing in the world, because the Cleveland Browns exist."

Miami Dolphins

A terrible team, gross colors, but people from Miami usually have drugs and are down to do stuff sexually.

Back to the nonsports options.

The Fez

Drives the quirk rating up; in a pinch can be used to bake a cake. Best when paired with a monkey in matching Fez and sunglasses.

The Sombrero

Dollar per square foot, you won't find more bang for your buck or pop for your peso than a sombrero. It always puts a smile on people's faces, unless they're racist. A sombrero is also fun because it inspires people to get drunk and party. And if you're one of them liberals, don't worry—cultural appropriation is fine if it happens at a bar!

The Turban

Let people think you're a high-flying Saudi playboy willing to buy bottle service for all with your unlimited petrodollars. It's warm, snug, and there's plenty of room to keep spare keys. For those of us who constantly fall down, it also doubles as an elegant ersatz helmet. Fun tip: If you're wearing a turban and have a trip planned, get to the airport three weeks early.

The Fedora

The fedora tells people you're either a 1940s private eye or a high school jazz instructor in a predominantly Caucasian community. Good luck either saving the dame or getting some kid named Cody to hit all the changes in "Watermelon Man"!

The Rat Pack all used to wear fedoras. The hat lends itself nicely to a whole swinger persona, where you call women "broads," "chicks," and "birds," to compensate for the fact that you're not a real man who can fix stuff like your dad. Plus, Martin Luther King and Malcolm X both wore fedoras and look at how everything turned out for them! One tip: Never pay full price for a fedora. They can be found very cheap in thrift stores, since almost everyone who ever owned one either died or their wife made them give it away.

The Toque

Say you're not only bald, but you're also the size of a ten-year-old? Lighter than a fireman's helmet and so inexpensive you can literally throw it away when you're done, the chef's hat—or toque—cleverly disguises baldness while adding a foot of height. It's not your fault your mother didn't breastfeed you and now you're five feet one. So why not hide all of your physical faults behind a fake passion for food?

Even though you're not allowed to eat, women will still find it attractive that you can prepare snacks, and you'll have a convenient reason to always be in the kitchen, hiding, at family events. You'll have to emerge with something, though, so here's an easy recipe for salmon that will make it appear you're not just dicking around in there.

SALMON TERIYAKI RECIPE

1. Get piece of salmon that's small enough to fit in oven. It doesn't need to be that fresh—you're not going to have any.
2. Spray pan with Pam, then place salmon in Pam pan.
3. Get bottle of teriyaki sauce and dump it all over salmon.
4. Broil salmon until top is blackened.
5. Turn off broiler, cook salmon at 350 degrees until internal temperature reaches 135.
6. Cut and serve to ungrateful family. If they don't like it, call them "Philistines!", break a window, and get profiled by *Vice* as "Cuisine's punk rock enfant terrible."

The Kangol

You can't dabble in the Kangol, it's a way of life, like diabetes or Scientology. If you wear it once, you have to become a "Kangol guy" and wear it forever, like Samuel L. Jackson. It's basically the herpes of hats. Kangols are cool, but you have to ask yourself, "Am I really *that* into kangaroos?"

The Beret

A beret is a great way to broadcast that you're French and uncircumcised. I advise against the beret because it looks like your hat just lost its erection.

Shoes

A subset of the hats category is shoes, which, if you think about it, are really just hats for your feet. A great pair of shoes completely flips the baldness paradigm: Don't look up at my head, look down here! In fact, painting two eyeballs, a nose, a mouth, and even hair on your shoes is enough to fool most people (they are probably buried in their phones anyway).

As you're deciding which hat will convey your entire identity going forward, it's time to learn the one, cardinal rule about social media: Bald men must never, ever, ever post a picture of their uncovered head on the Internet. If you're not in a hat, only post food, sunsets, and feet on a beach. Conveniently, you don't need to go anywhere, just swipe other people's sunsets, food, and feet and use them as your own. No one can prove that's not your tamale or toes. Here are a few examples from my great social media feed:

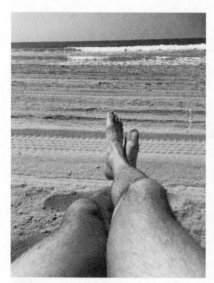

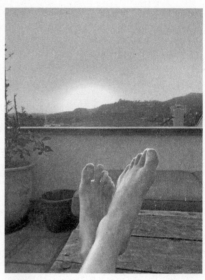

 Beachin' it! #swimfan

 Sunset funset! #nightfan

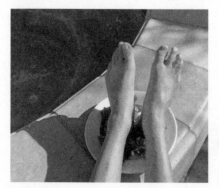

 Eatin' it, feetin' it! #foodfan

Simple, positive statements from an out-of-frame guy with feet who we can only assume also has hair. Several more photos are available on my website, verybald.com, with pre-written captions. Just be very careful your bald shadow never enters the picture or your whole life is blown.

Why not just be honest and show your head? Well, because then everyone everywhere in the world—from potential employers to blind dates—can search you and know you're bald. Then they won't hire you or boink you or both. You don't want anyone learning that information until you're at the interview or the sex and it's too late to do anything about it. Then when they say "I didn't realize you were bald," say "Neither did I" and continue interviewing or boinking, or both.

Believe it or not, you now know just as much as Albert Einstein did about hats, and you're well on your way to a powerful personal transformation. Because wearing a hat is like holding a poker hand—no one knows what you're hiding from them. Bald? Hair? They won't have a clue. You know it's a pair of twos, but maybe you can bluff people into thinking it's a royal flush (Jheri curl). Oh, one thing I should have mentioned earlier: You can never take that hat off ever again, even while you sleep. Okay, great!

Now we'll turn our attention from the top of your head to the middle of it, or, as we will refer to it from this point forward, your "face."

8

Glasses

Glasses are the single most distracting thing you can put on your face. Perhaps your vision is good so you don't need glasses? Then go outside and stare at the sun for thirty seconds. Congratulations, you now need glasses.

I own twelve pairs of glasses. I'm not kidding, here they are.

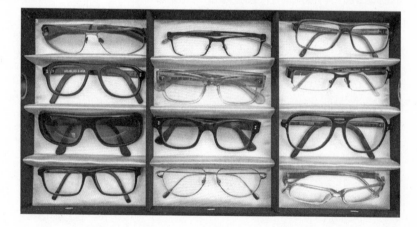

I basically have an optometrist's shop in my bedroom. All I need is a poster with a bunch of backward E's and I can start lecturing young people about glaucoma.

Glasses are incredibly useful for your image. They project that you're smarter than the person you're talking to, which makes them feel stupid and vulnerable. Simply by changing your spectacles, you can convince the world you're an entirely different type of person. I'll walk you through my pairs and the thought process behind them to illustrate their versatility.

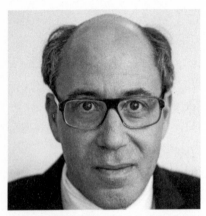

I call this one "guy who posed as a child molester to catch a child molester." He's a hero alright, but his portrayal of a child molester (that he used to catch a child molester!) was too convincingly creepy. No good deed goes unpunished. Anyway, keep him away from those Cub Scouts.

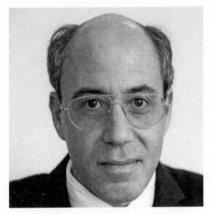

These have transition lenses. If I can make my glasses turn into sunglasses just by walking outside, imagine what else I can do! I'm a human Transformer! Or am I a Decepticon?! There's only one way to find out—spend hours trying to fold me!

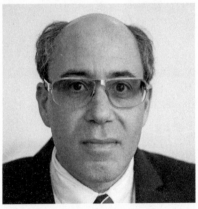

Remember 1999? This guy does. Playing Pokémon, cheering on Lance Armstrong, and Livin' La Vida Loca? Schwing!!! He owns thousands of shares of Enron and he'll let you know on Myspace if he survived Y2K.

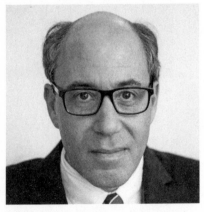

Allow me to show you various cheap caskets for your aunt.

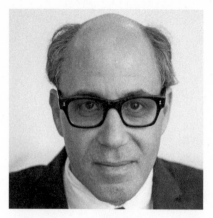

With this pair, you at least have to entertain the possibility I'm Jason Statham, which is the best thing a bald guy can be. I'm probably not Jason Statham because why would he be changing a baby's diaper in a gas station bathroom? But if I am, I can kick your ass in this gas station bathroom. Let's hope that during our fight that diaper stays where it is.

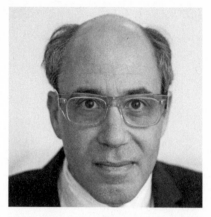

Hi, I'm the guy Zoe flies to San Francisco to buy pills from.

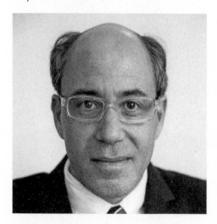

These are very specific, but when I need them, there's no substitute. It's "racquetball coach who makes a pass at you." We're in that racquetball court, working up a sweat, bodies are flying around, I know you felt the same chemistry I did. You didn't? Okay, the score is 11–7, let's keep playing.

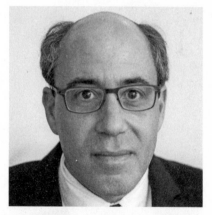

This attorney is the only person in the world who believes your wife fell down the stairs. He knows that just because you were having an affair with a man doesn't mean you committed murder. His retainer is $50,000 a month and he'll lose the case, but don't worry, he'll participate in the documentary that gets you a retrial (which he also loses).

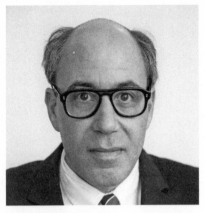

The thick black plastic ones were great until everyone kind of woke up at once to the fact that Woody Allen marrying his stepdaughter was probably wrong. Now they're kind of a "stay-away."

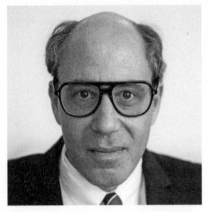

These are so ironic, they're unironic. My face is a hipster riddle. Am I trying to look stupid? Or am I so intentionally trying to look stupid that it's rad. I think they're cool, even if I have to turn sideways to get through doorways.

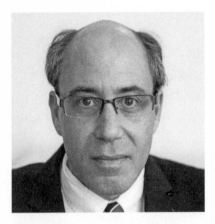

Wire frames are an elegant choice. They tell other people that you're an architect, without spending $200,000 for an actual degree. The ruse is easy to keep up; simply say stuff like "I think a bathroom would be good here," or "Oh, as an architect I recognize that's a bedroom." No one will expect you to do real work—contractors do all that. And no one will mistake you for a contractor, because you have glasses like a nerd.

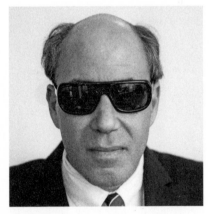

The Bono—this almost sixty-year-old, five-foot-one rocker still has a couple moves left in him! I still haven't found what I'm looking for! (A step stool so I can reach the pancake batter on the top shelf.)

Eye Patch

Technically the opposite of glasses, but nothing creates intrigue quite like the possibility of a missing eye. Without an eye patch, you're just a bald, boring two-eyed Joe. But with an eye patch, you'll become the subject of obsessive speculation: "Did he fall on a stick? Is he a pirate? Owl attack? Is he Zorro? Does he have a dark, secret past? Or did it happen, like, yesterday?"

People will hang on your every word, hoping you'll reveal what the heck knocked out your eyeball. Never get specific, but every once in a while, maybe mutter about a whale who wronged you. Men will want to be your friend, and women will throw themselves at you, or vice versa. Literally anything you draw on a napkin will be mistaken for a treasure map and send people off on a lifelong wild-goose chase.

I wear an eye patch to formal occasions like baptisms and weddings. It's a fantastic way to steal focus from people on their special day. A hook on the arm is also a nice touch, not to mention great for holding hamburgers. If security at the event says you're taking too many hamburgers, unsheathe your scabbard and challenge them to a duel. There's a 90 percent chance they'll back down, but if they accept, remove the eye patch. Otherwise, you'll be sword fighting with no depth perception. (On the other hand, if they stab you in the eye— eye patch!)

9

Facial Hair

Like the earth itself, your face is full of unused real estate. For land to be worth anything you need to build on it. Growing a mustache is sort of like building condos under your nose. At first, people may point and ask, "Why is that there? This neighborhood sucks and it's far away from everything. It's a forty-minute train ride to the ears." Eventually, though, artists will move in, microbreweries will crop up, and young bohemians will begin to realize "Hey, this area is pretty hip. I can't afford anything here, therefore I will live here." Before you know it, your mustache and beard can be the cool Brooklyn to the lame Manhattan of your bald head.

Facial hair psychologically fulfills a huge need. It allows you to get back on that hair horse after you've fallen off and it's trampled you. It may not be exactly where you want it, but it's hair you can cut, grow, and style. And the mustache has several other virtues. It gives you something to twist while you're solving mysteries. It's visual proof you've hit puberty and should be allowed to watch PG-13 movies. It provides a sanctuary for all the lice refugees driven from your head.

Plus, grow a mustache and you can now wear one of those hilarious "Mustache Rides, 25 Cents" baseball caps!

A brief digression on the economic model of mustache rides: The price is appallingly low and it's killing suppliers. It hasn't risen from 25 cents in decades. I've even seen hats and t-shirts offering mustache rides for as low as 5 cents, or even free!

Given the high cost of waxes, pomades, and postride face maintenance, there's no path to profitability at 5 or even 25 cents per ride, even in a high-volume business. The mustache owner hemorrhages over $4 per ride, despite virtually no customer acquisition cost from the hat. As you burn runway at an alarming rate, good luck attracting a B-round of financing—you've undoubtedly given up way too much equity too soon and scared off investors.

I guarantee if you showed up on *Shark Tank* offering twenty-five-cent mustache rides, Lori and Daymond would go out immediately. Robert would say he loves the idea, but he's a customer, not a partner. Mark would pound you on the fundamentals, and point out there's nothing proprietary about people sitting on your face. Barbara would be mad she was clearly your last choice. Finally, Mr. Wonderful would offer you a loan at 15 percent but want a royalty of 20 cents per ride in perpetuity, which you will turn down because he's a hairless amoral snake. You will leave without a deal.

That's why if you're going to offer mustache rides, I propose a revolutionary new fee structure: Annual membership at $300 a year.

Like those who join a gym, most people committing to a year-long contract of mustache rides will only show up for a "'stache bash" on New Year's Day. But say for the sake of argument they want ten rides a year. At $300 (Incredible deal! Less than a dollar a day!) you're still amortizing m-rides at $30 a literal pop. Now, suddenly, you have enough money to rent a small gallery where you give the mustache rides instead of squatting in the alley behind TJ Maxx.

Who cares if you get underpriced by the competition? Who's

going to look more professional? You, in a gallery? Or a bald guy wearing a hat who wants to lick vaginas for a nickel?

A switch to a yearly mustache ride membership model could be a real boon to the economy, providing steady union jobs for real American workers.

So I ask that all bald men immediately stop wearing hats that say "Mustache Rides, 25 Cents" and instead wear the hat "Mustache Rides, $300 Annual Membership Fee" available on my website, verybald.com.

Let's stop being idiots and start being properly paid for cunnilingus. Thank you.

Here are several mustaches and beards to choose from, ranging from beginner to extremely advanced. You may want to consult your doctor before growing any facial hair, because he's a control freak and the last thing you want to do is make him angry. If you're in a real hurry, any of the following can just be drawn on with a Sharpie.

The Selleck

The greater the distance between your mouth and nose, the more impressive this mustache is. Tom Selleck himself has an epic eight-mile gap. To put that in perspective, more than seven thousand people can lie head to toe between Tom Selleck's lips and nostrils, a feat once verified on the set of *Blue Bloods*. Beware: This mustache may become sentient, drain your bank account, and move to Hawaii.

The Drifter/Wizard

Popularized by David Letterman, this is an attempt to show you've "given up" and have transcended any concerns related to appearance. Downside: Get ready to be called "Dumblebald."

The Hair Pie

A long beard is smashed into a piping hot blueberry pie, creating a crumble that hardens into the beard as it cools and gives it flavor. The beard may then be used as a dessert lick where people come up and suck on the ends.

The Elfio

This is a facial hair configuration I invented. The whiskers are grown for years, split, then pulled behind the ears and under the chin, where they meet and are then tied into a festive bow, creating a wonderful holiday mustache.

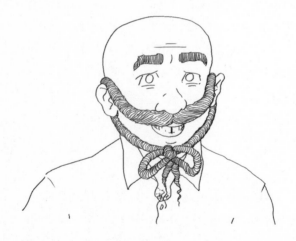

The Stachotard

Developed in the famed Swedish mustache lab of Frstbrüg, the beard is grown to floor length, then pulled through the crotch, channeled through the anus crack, up the back, then duct-taped to the top of the shoulders, like a hair leotard. It's basically a completely legal way to be naked in public. It does nothing for you socially, as people will assume you're crazy. However, it's quite comfortable for alpine bathing and provides a natural cushion when sitting on a granite boulder and playing your harp.

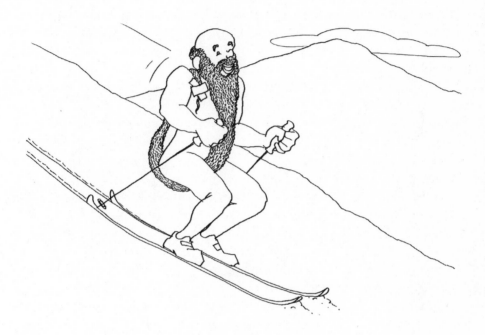

Things are rapidly changing in the world of mustaches and beards, and I'm beyond excited to tell you about a new innovation: the multiperson intertwining facial hair project. This is when you pair up with other bald men and turn yourselves into a living piece of facial art. In India, people are doing things with three-, four-, and even five-person mustaches that were impossible even a few years ago. The technology is so recent that the ideas that follow come with the caveat that long-term effects are unknown. Here are a few standout ideas from this new, burgeoning field.

The Jump Rope

The world's first two-person mustache. Each party grows one side long, and the two are then tied together with either a running bowline knot or a sheepshank. The conjoined mustaches then provide a rope for children to engage in double Dutch. Please note: It may be difficult to find parents willing to let their children participate.

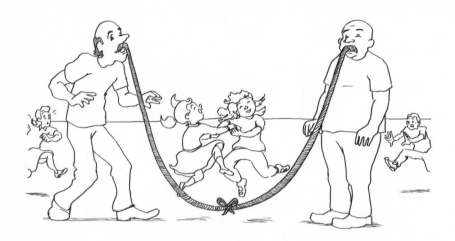

The Human Stachipede

The mustache of the person in the rear is tied into the mustache of the person in the front, securing their two bodies together with facial hair, allowing the caboose to eat the feces of the engine. The engine can eat regular food. I haven't tried this.

(Image redacted.)

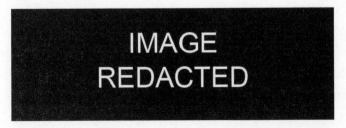

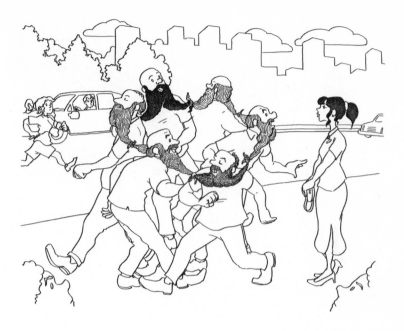

The Carousel

Four or more bald men grow long beards, split them, and tie the ends together. An equal number face inward and outward, so moving forward or backward becomes less efficient. This encourages a return to a simple time of "slow living." Carousels can work for groups of even a hundred bald men or more, creating a sort of "bald man rat king." Women can "speed date" the entire carousel by walking around and talking to each member at her leisure.

Housetaches and Roof Wigs

(Utility patent pending.) These are giant prosthetics you mount on your domicile to give your house a full head of hair and/or a mustache. Your house now looks like a cool guy you'd talk to at a bar, and you, in effect, have hair—not on your head, but over your head on your roof. Your house will be the talk of your street and probably the subject of several contentious town hall meetings!

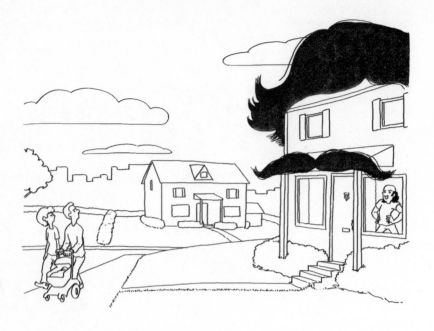

Fair warning: There have been anecdotal reports of the first production batch of roof wigs retaining water during hurricanes and blizzards, causing roofs to collapse and crush sleeping families. The kinks are still being worked out, and once we land on a new polymer, the old unsafe ones will be available on my website at a steep discount.

Skeptical that beards, weird clothing, and a hat won't work? Check out this guy:

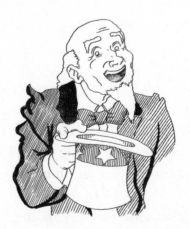

That's right, Uncle Sam is bald, and you never noticed until this very second! His star-spangled get-up, flag waving, and enthusiastic pointing have put everyone off the scent for over two hundred years. He immediately throws everyone he encounters on the defensive by demanding they join the army. They're so scared of looking like hippie chickenshits, they fail to investigate his whole hair sitch. You should adopt this approach. Upon encountering anyone with hair, promptly accuse them of treason. Let them disprove your accusations by enlisting and going off to war. With all the men with hair off fighting overseas, bald guys get their pick of the ladies! That's smart bald thinking, and the patriotic power of personality.

You've now had a completely comprehensive master class in personal transformation. You're ready to deceive others, but more important, you're ready to deceive yourself. Obviously, the only limits are your creativity and the size of the loan a bank will give you for glasses. If one persona doesn't work, simply leave those jackets/hats/gold chains/goggles by the ocean for some other bald guy to take and try something else. If you have a monocle, sombrero, Yosemite Sam mustache, vampire fangs, and are riding a kiteboard with a baby tiger, surely *somebody* will want to hang out with you.

If all else fails, start with the basics: goatee, neck tattoo, diamond chin ring, and cargo shorts. Greet everyone with "You good?" and people will assume you're a drug dealer. Suddenly, people at bars and clubs who would never even look at you before will approach, begging to know what you have. If you can actually sell them some drugs, so much the better. Now you have customers, and any decent salesman with angel dust can turn customers into friends.

Without much effort, you'll suddenly have a bunch of addicts depending on you, employees plotting against you, women using you, rival dealers trying to kill you—in other words, *you've built a life.*

Say you get convicted of a felony? Well, that's fantastic! You'll be legally prohibited from voting, so you never have to watch the news again!

But what if all this is too much for you? What if you'd rather just go back to having hair? Let's explore all the unsatisfactory ways you can do that in "Plugs, Drugs, and Rugs"!

10

Plugs, Drugs, and Rugs

How is it you can walk into any Walmart and buy a gun, then walk into Planned Parenthood and get an abortion—basically, have a full, awesome day—but you can't walk into a hospital and get your old hair back? It's a good question, and one you should tweet constantly from your company's account.

The good news is, scientists are at work on the problem. The bad news is, like floating cars, moving sidewalks, or a cell-phone that makes clear calls, promising developments always seem just around the corner, then never appear. Frankly, between tantric bald-solving and failing at cancer, these manipulative science geeks are making a fortune pretending to pour stuff into test tubes. They know we would pay anything for a bald cure, so they keep saying they're about to find one, so we keep giving them money. Meanwhile, they're laughing all the way to the lab.

It seems like every few weeks you hear that something "works on mice." Here's the deep, dark secret, though: Everything works on mice! Their life expectancy is only two years, so literally any substance will give them a few extra days.

Lab mice are having the time of their lives right now, running around thin, cancer-free, and with gorgeous manes of hair. We've basically spent billions creating a race of rodent Bradley Coopers.

If there was a surefire cure for baldness, it would be available, because all of us would spend all our money for it. Jeff Bezos would look like Russell Brand. No Jew would be bald. I mean, we control the *weather* for God's sake. (I know that sounds insane, but I swear, right after my bar mitzvah, I was whisked into a room that looked like a cross between a 1970s newsroom and a matzoh factory, where I briefly shook hands with George Soros. He gave me a joystick to manipulate, which caused it to rain in Mobile, Alabama. The whole thing took less than three minutes and was a lot less fun than it sounds.)

If there was a solution to baldness, you wouldn't have to skulk around on weird websites—you'd know about it. It's like how cocaine doesn't need to advertise. We all know it's there and our stockbroker friend, Joey, has some. But we also know that if we want the cocaine, we have to hang out with Joey, who will ruin all the fun of being on cocaine. That's the baldness remedy conundrum in a nutshell. Everything comes at a cost, financial, emotional, or erectile, that I'm not sure I'm willing to pay.

All that said, like medieval prisoners given a choice between death by hanging, flaying, or being burned alive at the stake, you nevertheless have several options when it comes to hair replacement.

Surgery

If you opt for hair-transplant surgery, the first thing you will need to do is choose a surgeon. If you're like me, you'll want to see a picture of the surgeon to see if he has hair. After a while, you will realize you've spent several months looking at—and judging—the hotness of thousands of surgeons. None of these surgeons will be female and many will look like guys you remember telling you dirty jokes when your dad took you to a junkyard to get parts for his old Saab.

You'll make an appointment and think about canceling it every ten seconds for the next few weeks. Then you'll drive to the clinic and have a meltdown in your car. You'll look around and make disconcerting eye contact with another bald man having a meltdown in his car. He'll speed off, burning rubber, ironically balding his tires.

You'll get into the doctor's office and have several minutes to ponder that you, a bald man, are waiting for someone to tell you if they'll take thousands of dollars to give you hair. Finally, he'll barge into the room, you'll exchange a few pleasantries, and he'll tell you, "Put your pants on, I'm not that kind of doctor."

You'll sit while he examines your head and makes a bunch of weird noises. Each noise will make you fear more and more that he's just discovered you have cancer and the appointment is about to go completely sideways.

You'll then be evaluated according to the Norwood Scale of Baldness.

The so-called Norwood Scale measures degrees of baldness so you and your plastic surgeon can avoid phrases like "You have kind of a circle thingy on top and wisps up front," or "Your head looks like it was eaten by moths."

Hey, Norwood, thank you so much for depicting the individual gradations of dignity loss in one place. The man in the poster's life is falling apart, but I guess it's all a big profitable joke to you! I hope your house gets infested by bats! (Note: If you hate this chart, you should *not* look at his poster of penis sizes.)

Anyway, how is this chart not a hate crime? Would we accept a poster detailing levels of "boob sagginess" or "lardassity"? I repudiate this chart, because I believe that just as every snowflake is unique, every bald man is hairless in his own beautiful way. I will not be reduced to a number! (Only because I'm a "seven." Honestly, if I was a "one" I'd be totally fine with it.)

The purpose, of course, is to find your counterpart on the chart, a sort of "show me where the bad man touched you" of baldness. Here's what each stage *really* means.

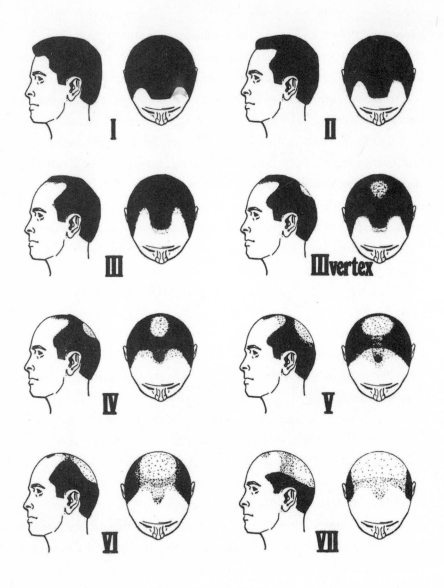

Stage One

"Hey man, everything's cool. Maybe there's a little thinness up front? Who knows, I'm more excited about my band. We're playing the Viper Room on Tuesday. I can't get you on the list, but you should come."

Stage Two

"Turns out no one goes to the Viper Room on Tuesdays. Mike's uncle, who worked for the label, lost his job. Not that labels are even really a thing anymore, I mean—everything is streaming now. And yeah, I may have lost a few more hairs, but I have bigger problems. Rent is due on the tenth, bro."

Stage Three

"Can you help me move? You won't have to move my drums, I pawned those. I'm gonna crash with my parents for a bit while I get my next thing off the ground. Mike and I think maybe instead of a band, we should start a company that makes rolling papers with Jack Black's face on them."

Stage Four

"Jack Black's suing us, man! How uncool is that??!"

Stage Five

"Constance dumped me! She said she can't be with some drummer who's not even in a band! We've been going out seven years! I've only been with one other woman! Now I'm supposed to hit the dating market when I'm twenty-nine, Norwood-stage-five bald, and owe Jack Black ten million dollars?"

Stages Six and Seven

There's nothing for stages six and seven because he blew his brains out.

Could it be coincidence that there are seven levels of baldness?

Just as there are seven levels on the Bristol Stool Scale for bowel health?

Bristol Stool Scale

Type 1		Separate hard lumps, like nuts, hard to pass
Type 2		Sausage-shaped, but lumpy
Type 3		Like a sausage, but with cracks on its surface
Type 4		Like a sausage or a snake, smooth and soft
Type 5		Soft blobs with clear-cut edges, passed easily
Type 6		Fluffy pieces with ragged edges, a mushy stool
Type 7		Watery, no solid pieces. Entirely liquid

Goal Stool Types

© Alila Medical Media - *www.AlilaMedicalMedia.com*

It got me thinking that these two charts could be combined for some good toupee variations.

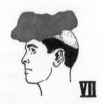

"I'm a seven, just diarrhea on my head."

Here I should point out, the term "hair transplant" is a misnomer for the surgery that actually occurs. A transplant implies that someone dies, a bunch of their body is stuffed into an Igloo cooler, then you get their cool, mostly unused parts and emerge from surgery a handsome two-human Frankenstein.

What really happens is *you* take hair from your *own* head and move it to a different part of your own head. (Motorcycle accident optional.)

After learning this, fatal motorcycle accidents were no longer the joyous occasions I thought they were. I used to pass them, thinking, "Sweet, someone's gonna get that guy's hair," and give everyone standing around in shock the "thumbs-up." But now that I understand more, motorcycle accidents just seem like tragic (but still, cool) wastes of life.

There are two types of hair-transplant surgery, F.U.E. and F.U.T. It's never a good sign when both of your options begin with "F.U." You can see the results of each by going to bald message boards and looking at the pictures of the tops of guys' heads who live in Indonesia.

The distinction between the two techniques is how and where you're getting your donor hair. With F.U.T. (Follicular Unit Transplant), strips of follicles are taken off the back of your neck, then transplanted onto your bald spot. The procedure leaves a scar where the strips were, so now both sides of your head look like shit. It's cheaper than F.U.E., but maybe hair restoration is a place you shouldn't be looking to save money, you know, like parachutes?

F.U.E. (Follicular Unit Extraction) takes thousands of individual follicles from the back and transplants them to the front. Sure, maybe it's rearranging deck chairs on the *Titanic*, but even if the boat's sinking, it must have felt good to finally have those chairs in the right place for the last twenty minutes. Supposedly, *Titanic* captain Edward J. Smith's last words were "Yeah, that actually really improves the flow."

Instead of one linear scar, F.U.E. leaves thousands of tiny dot scars, which will rain down a week or two later in a dry scab hurricane. With either procedure, the less bald you are, the better it works. For it to be most effective, you need to act immediately when you think you might be going bald and combine it with drug therapy. Which means the baldest men who need it the most—like me—stand to benefit the least. At best, I can pay ten grand to maybe go back to the receding hairline that bummed me out in the first place.

Which begs the obvious question: Why not leave all the hair where it is, drill new holes for your eyeballs in the back of your head, transplant your eyes, nose, and mouth and make the back of your head the front? Unfortunately, my doctor said it's not feasible at this time, although they've successfully done it to mice, because of course they have.

I also asked the doctor about the possibility of transplanting thousands of pubes up onto my head, and he told me to leave his mother's funeral.

Surgery is a huge emotional and financial commitment, so you should come prepared with important questions to ask your doctor, such as:

- Which technique do you use and why?
- What's your postoperation protocol to ensure against infection?
- Where did you go to medical school, you butcher?
- For an extra $10, will you touch me without gloves?
- Will the anesthetic be general or local, and what do you anticipate the recovery challenges will be?
- Which of your kids do you love the most and why?
- Are lab coats white so they can hide semen?
- How soon will I be able to jet-ski after the procedure? Anything longer than nine minutes is unacceptable.

In my case, I wasn't personally ready to commit to the surgery. I thought of friends who'd had teeth whitened. It never made them look better. It just made parts of them I'd never noticed before now look worse by comparison. That's the problem with fixing anything—put a brand-spanking-new door on your 1998 Chrysler, and it actually draws more attention to how bad the rest of the car looks.

In the end, I stumbled on a rather elegant compromise: I have a hair on my boob that grows long incredibly fast. It is absolutely the star follicle on my body. I keep trimming it, because it makes my nipple look like one of Betty Boop's eyes, but it keeps growing back, stronger and more determined than before. This follicle is truly the most glorious thing about me and teaches me a daily lesson about the indomitability of the human spirit.

And after several rounds of pleading, the doctor agreed to transplant it onto my head.

It's just one hair, but in my darkest moments, when I feel beyond redemption, I can stroke it, cradle it, turn to it as a sign that all hope is not lost. Even in the most barren desert, a single rose can arise. And if one rose can rise, why not hundreds? And if hundreds, why not thousands? And why couldn't a new era of peace and—

Oops, it just fell out.

11

Drugs!

Let's start with the good news: You've finally decided to do something! Good for you!

The bad news: It's already too late!

Most of the drug options won't grow new hair; they'll simply help you preserve what you already have. If you're freaked out about how little hair you've got, drugs probably aren't the answer. Typical of bald life, your worst-case scenario may suddenly be the best option. I mean, the single good thing you can say about balding is at least it's free. Drugs, shampoos, and lotions can cost hundreds of dollars a month just to maintain the status quo that has you in a spiral.

Here are a few of the lovingly hand-crafted local artisanal medications you can try.

Minoxidil, aka Rogaine

Minoxidil comes in either a foam, a shampoo, or a conditioner. It's the only over-the-counter drug approved by the FDA for hair loss. Supposedly, it's best for dudes who are at the beginning stages of balding and may help you retain and even grow a bit of hair.

Without getting overly technical, minoxidil works by you rubbing it in, then praying you see something. If you don't, the fault is with your stupid head and not their amazing drug.

Minoxidil costs around $50 a month, and of course, the second you stop using it, all your new hair may fall out, so congratulations, you're now hostage to a foam.

Shampoos

There are various antibaldness shampoos sold online, but I found they all have one thing in common: They don't work. And I'll admit I was shocked. Until very recently, I thought everything I read online was true. But it turns out no one's, like, checking.

The honest shampoos will say they don't regrow hair, they preserve and thicken what you already have. If you have hair that's capable of being preserved and thickened, well then, la-di-da for you, you bald poseur. My head is a parched *Mad Max* wasteland that's suitable only for motocross enduro racing and boron mining. Still, I gave it a go. And in all fairness, several coworkers did say my back hair looked especially lustrous, before my boss told me to put my shirt on and gave me a stern "final warning."

Keep in mind the root of the word "shampoo" is the Latin *sham* meaning "sham" and *poo* meaning "shit," so literally, shampoo is "fakeshit." I did find one shampoo online that claimed to regrow my hair, but its claims were not substantiated by the FDA. This was fine by me—I mistrust the government and think they hide all the good drugs from us like crank and acid, so I was ready to send the makers $300 a month.

I know what you're thinking, "Three hundred dollars a month?! That's a crapload of money!" It's the equivalent of buying two pairs of True Religion jeans, which are basically a toupee for your ass! You could give $150 a month to the American Red Cross and still have enough left over to give $150 to the armed rebels who are causing the crisis! You could buy a plane ticket to Toronto *and* a gorilla costume to wear on the flight!

I gave the shampoo a whirl. It smelled good and foamed up nicely. Like most shampoos, if you jerk off with it, it burns your pee-hole, but they don't tell you that on the website, believe you me. I have been battling with the FDA for years to put a giant warning on every bottle of shampoo sold, but clearly the Feds are more concerned with corporate profits than your stinging pee-hole. (Conditioner works fine.)

Ten minutes after washing it off (my head), I didn't notice much growth, but later it did create tons of bubbles when I poured it into a hotel fountain and sent all the employees into a panic, so I feel like I got my money's worth. Definitely get some and pour it into a hotel fountain.

Propecia

Propecia began as a prostate drug, then doctors noticed an interesting phenomenon—all these old baldies who couldn't pee were suddenly regrowing hair. It was then Propecia took on a second life as a hair-loss drug. And it does regrow hair for a lot of people.

However, like any wonder drug, Propecia lists a bunch of side effects apart from hair growth. "Headache, dizziness, nausea." Okay, I don't remember the last time I didn't have those. I've been hungover since 1993. "Depression and thoughts of suicide." Forget side effects, those are the main effects of baldness, so no additional risk there! "Scaly nipples and nipple discharge." Well, now you're talking me into it! And . . . "impotence."

Oh boy.

We're now at the crux of the essential dilemma of hair loss: Which would you rather be, a bald guy with a boner, or some limp dick with hair? What a horrible "Sophie's choice" we are locked into, forced to pick either hair or boners. How to decide? Let's turn to one of history's great thinkers.

When former Secretary of Defense Donald Rumsfeld was conceiving his brilliant invasion of Iraq, he thought in terms of "known knowns," "known unknowns," and "unknown unknowns."

To me the known knowns are: I like having boners and it sucks not having hair. The known unknowns are: Could the Propecia cause me to lose my boners or shoot geysers from my nips? Will nothing happen? Could I achieve the best outcome of having hair, boners, and nipple bazookas? The unknown unknowns are, of course, unknowable.

I've never lived without boners, but I have lived without hair. Once you go bald, there is a certain comfort in knowing it can't get worse. It's not like your head starts peeling off and you're walking around with an exposed brain. I would have loved more information about living without boners but getting people to talk about impotence is (ironically) harder (get it?) than engaging them to talk about baldness. In the end, in spite of approaching thousands of men with their families at a carnival and asking if they're impotent, I didn't get a single "yes."

I simply can't imagine exchanging pleasure for appearance. Just as cutting the arts during wartime raises the question "What are we fighting for?" if you can't get erections, why do you need hair?

If you already can't get erections, I highly recommend Propecia because what else do you have to lose? You might as well try to get some fuzz going. And maybe you'd luck out and not have the side effects. But is that really the kind of luck you have? You're already bald! I know I'd get the side effects. I'm unlucky and mistime everything. My second day of college, Magic Johnson said he had AIDS and no one had sex for two years. I bought AOL right before it crashed. I left a job at *Family Guy* to write on the show *Dads*. If you want to double down and roll the erection dice, go right ahead. I'd rather cash in my chips and live to play another day at the ChubHub Casino.

However, I've saved the best for last. There is one surefire, no-joke cure for baldness that has been tested and proved to work.

Castration

By cutting off your nut sack, testosterone production stops, so your hair never falls out.

Getting someone to agree to castrate you, though, is difficult. I called the front desk at Cedars Sinai Hospital several times asking them to connect me with their castration department and was hung up on immediately. I decided I needed to go right to the top, so I dialed 911. No one would help, and they were all in a huge hurry to get off the phone. Very rude.

Then I realized, castration is something you can do at home. I relaxed, put on Stevie Wonder's *Musiquarium I, Volume 2*, and profoundly iced my balls. Once they were good and numb, I sharpened my fanciest Japanese katana, placed my nuts on a sturdy Boos block cutting board, and raised the blade above my head. As I was about to Benihana my ballbag, I caught a glimpse of my reflection in the living room window: A naked bald man holding an heirloom warrior knife to his own testicles. "What are you doing?" I shrieked.

In shock, I dropped the katana, then noticed my mailman staring at me through the window, wearing his stupid summer shorts and pith helmet. "G'way! G'way!" I shouted, then shooed him off my stoop with a broom. Terrified, he threw a Valpak at me, then scurried off. I stumbled back inside, naked, shocked, spent, then collapsed on the floor.

My dog looked down at me unsympathetically as if to say, "You cut off mine. Now all of a sudden you get morals?"

The Laser Helmet

Every man remembers three days in his life: the day he learns to drive, the day he loses his virginity, and the day he gets his laser hair-growth helmet.

The helmet, unlike many of those foams and creams, *is* an FDA-approved baldness remedy. Most of these helmets were so expensive,

I'd written off having one. Then, one day, I was sitting at my desk deciding between paying some bills or spending nine hours watching pornography when an email showed up in my spam folder—a Groupon offer for laser helmets! Finally, bald men were working together, harnessing their purchasing power to drive down the cost of this wholly necessary item. My laser helmet cost $450, which seemed cheap for something that has a ton of lasers in it.

(I only wish I could meet the other men who participated in the laser helmet Groupon. I'd love to become best friends and take yearly vacations and come up with a fun name for ourselves like "the Alan Baldas." If you're out there, please contact me. I'm totally willing to abandon my family for this.)

I have to admit to some preliminary confusion about laser hats. After all, walking around Los Angeles, where I live, you see hundreds of places for laser hair removal, because I guess a lot of people are looking inside other people's butts and judging. So lasers eliminate hair, right? Well, not so fast. Because this made-in-China thing with instructions that may have been written by a human slave says that lasers grow hair. Which is it? How can it be both? Is it possible that lasers kill some hairs but grow others, with the net result being a slight percentage increase? Or would numerous hairless Los Angeles upper lips and judged butts beg to differ?

I tested the helmet on my baby for a month and thought it worked amazingly well, then realized she was naturally growing hair anyway. I hope it has no lasting long-term effects, but too late to stuff that cat back in the bag. After a while, sitting there for thirty minutes every day wearing this thing got very boring, so I synced it up to some EDM, ate a weed brownie, and had my own laser-light hair show, which was pretty mind-blowing. It made me realize: We are all two.

We associate wearing a helmet indoors with mental impairment, so it didn't really help my image to have it on at work, except on the day the fire alarm sounded and I was able to function as an emergency beacon and lead people out to a predesignated meeting point.

I noticed they sent the bald fireman in to battle the blaze, while two guys with hair worked the hose.

After months of investigating drugs, wearing helmets, drinking shampoos, and having nipple hairs put on my head, I concluded these "solutions" are all to some degree effective, though all are far from perfect. And while I can't read your mind, I predict you'll remain dissatisfied, and here's why: These remedies don't provide a permanent solution. Rather, they lock you into a state of perpetual balding—instead of ripping the Band-Aid off once and being done with it, you tear it off slightly more each day, prolonging your pain indefinitely. This is a kind of purgatory. Neither bald nor haired, neither fish nor fowl. You don't have nearly enough hair to compete with the haired, yet you're not bald enough to be in the clean pate club.

While surgery gives great results for some, it's not the end of the baldness process; it's a new beginning. Pattern baldness continues in spite of your transplants. You may find yourself needing a second or third surgery to play catch up, as you pile up Acme traps trying and failing to catch the elusive Road Runner of baldness.

Remember back when I talked about loss aversion, how the pain of losing something outweighs the pleasure of gaining the same? Regardless of the option you choose, you will still be losing hair, daily, monthly, yearly, and the agony from loss aversion will grow and grow. You'll be locked into a never-ending race with your own body to patch up the new leaks.

Second, and more significantly, you will always be comparing the results to yourself with your fullest head of hair, not you at your baldest. No matter how much hair you gain, you'll still experience a net loss vis-à-vis your conception of your ideal self, and this loss will feel worse than the gain of new hair.

Just as Shakespeare (bald) voiced through Julius Caesar (bald), "Cowards die many times before their death; the valiant never taste of death but once," I believe that people with hair transplants go bald many times, whereas those who do nothing go bald only once.

In fact, the entire play *Julius Caesar* is a searing allegory for baldness written by Shakespeare, a bald man. Cut through all the flowery language and the message is clear: It's okay for someone with hair to murder a bald guy in broad daylight as long as you name a salad dressing for him later.

I urge you to break this cycle, accept you're bald, and learn to cope from there. Then you can save your money and put it toward a guaranteed path to happiness: penis enlargement surgery.

Or, like me, having given plugs, drugs, helmets, and shampoo a completely unfair shake, you could seek out a more permanent temporary solution.

12

A Tale of Toupees

I think we all accept as a fact that toupees are ridiculous and those who wear them are buffoons. But why? Because a person has tried to replace what's missing with a substitute?

We don't make fun of people with a prosthetic leg. We'd never belittle someone with one of those face transplants. We only make fun of people missing fingers when we're drunk and are sure no one is filming us. Why should a toupee be mocked any more than the use of a wheelchair?

In fact, I would argue in light of "hair privilege," baldness *is* a kind of handicap. We're missing a part of our bodies that makes life easier.

I'm not saying bald people should be able to park in handicapped spots. I'm saying bald people should have a designated area in between handicapped and regular parking where we leave our cars. Then we wouldn't have to walk by people with hair on our way to the mall. We'd only pass people in wheelchairs, with whom we have a signed treaty to lay off each other.

These thoughts floated through my

head as I parked behind the toupee shop, grateful they had a back entrance, so I could shamefully army-crawl in. Once inside, the receptionist took my name and information, then tactfully asked what my budget was. "Six million dollars," I replied, so they wouldn't think I was some kind of small-town rube. Then I was led to a room with a barber's chair, a disconcerting number of mirrors, and zero cellphone reception.

Soon the door opened, and a slim, pretty, and cheerful Asian woman in her early sixties introduced herself as Joyce. I was nervous, ashamed, and babbling, feeling weird about even being there, and her whole demeanor instantly put me at ease. Joyce offered me tea, which I refused because I'm a guy. She then offered me water, which I turned down on the gamble she would then offer me some third, better thing. When she didn't, I felt stupid for not taking the water but realized asking for it after having refused it would make me look like some kind of maniac. So I stayed thirsty.

Joyce explained she'd made thousands of hair systems. She assured me the end product would be comfortable, look completely authentic, and be made of 100 percent human hair. She promised me that she wasn't going to stick a brown muskrat on my head in a futile attempt to make me appear twenty years old. She would create a realistic, age-appropriate hairline, even blending the gray, all to create a seamless, dignified, and, most important, realistic head of hair.

Joyce said there are thousands of options, then handed me one of those hairstyle books you used to see in 1980s barbershops. Everyone in the book looked like a mutant version of a celebrity, and it was easy to imagine each of these toupees leading to a new and distinct life.

There was a guy who looked like if Johnny Depp got trampled then smoothed out again. He wore a very intriguing amulet around his neck, as if to imply this hairstyle book might be a portal to deeper cosmic mysteries.

There was a guy who looked like if you bought John Krasinski from Ikea and he was missing a part but it was too long a drive to return him to the store, so you decided to assemble him anyway.

Then, in the middle of the book, there was just George Clooney— I can't believe they got him to do that. They must have paid a fortune for the rights.

So many potential futures! With the blond ponytail, I could live in the Alps with a stout lass named Helga and our two Norse sons, who can be a "handful" but are ultimately good kids.

With the Afro, I'm reincarnated as Malik el-Shabazz, a nightclub-owning Moroccan with a penchant for fast cars and even faster girls and even fastest guys.

Rocker . . . cool corporate guy . . . camp counselor who didn't quite molest you but did something wrong that you could never clearly articulate . . . they have 'em all.

Browsing the toupee choices, I felt like a starving man being released into a Las Vegas buffet. You have no idea what to eat first— crab legs, barbecue, pancakes, donuts? So you make a giant pile and devour it all, while the person across from you silently decides the relationship is over. I hadn't had hair in twenty years and I wanted to make up for lost time by gorging on everything at once: parts, ponytails, spikes, rat tails, bangs. In that moment, I became hair Caligula.

For the first time in as long as I could remember, I was excited about the unknown future. While I dreamed, Joyce took precise measurements of my head. She then wrapped my skull in Saran Wrap and began crafting a precise plaster cast to send to Thailand, where they'd manufacture my custom hairpiece with, again, 100 percent human hair. During this procedure, she significantly allayed my fears by answering questions such as:

- Do I need to get a Styrofoam head to store the toupee?

- Should I have a backup Styrofoam head in case my primary Styrofoam head is blown away in a gale?

- Do you sell separate eyes and mustaches for the Styrofoam head?

- Do the Styrofoam heads come in different races?

- Is "Ron" a good name for a Styrofoam head?

- What's the most number of questions anyone has ever asked about Styrofoam heads?

- Will the toupee make my head more flammable?

- Do I have to give up fireworks? Because I have a big shipment of fireworks coming.

- Do I need to wet the system down before I run into a burning building to save children?

- I like to dump bananas flambé on my head as a joke. Do I need to stop doing this?

- Does bird shit come out of this stuff or would I have to cut my head off?

Joyce told me that since the toupee is made from 100 percent human hair, you can light fireworks, run into burning buildings, and put toucans on your head, just like everybody does, with zero fear. Joyce finished her cast, told me she'd have my piece in four weeks, then deftly staved off my hug with a handshake.

As I drove home, I was struck by how the toupee, at its core, contains a fascinating dilemma: Is it better to be bald, or a liar? Each toupee is implicitly a lie. As we meet new people, we enter into an unspoken compact that we are who we say we are and who we appear. But especially in intimate relationships, the toupee requires eventual disclosure. Or does it?

Do we owe those whom we are dating (or even just fingering) the straight poop on our hair? If they can't tell, what harm is there in a lie? After all, there are many things that remain hidden even in the best relationships.

It also creates a fascinating paradox: If a person would have you without the toupee, then you don't need the toupee. But if they wouldn't want you sans rug, would you want to be with them anyway? (Of course you would.)

Many of the most famous celebrities pulled the wool over the eyes of a gullible America. John Wayne wore a toupee. No wonder he has resting bitch face in all his movies. Jimmy Stewart had a ru-ru-ru-rug. Bing Crosby found time in his famous beating-his-kids schedule to get fake hair.

Which brings us to Frank Sinatra. He had more than thirty toupees, but that's not even the shocking part.

I am going to let you in on the details of a conspiracy so vast and dangerous that my life may be in danger. Can I prove my theory? Not at all—but, can you disprove it? How do you know?—you haven't heard it yet. As they say, "Extraordinary claims require extraordinary disproof." So without further ado, here goes:

President Kennedy was assassinated because he was about to reveal Frank Sinatra was bald.

It's no secret that Frank Sinatra and Kennedy were friends. Kennedy spent time at Sinatra's legendary Palm Springs house, where the men had an endless appetite for two things: Yahtzee and broads. If they weren't throwing around the old dice and screaming "Yahtzee!" they were throwing around their old wieners and screaming "Yahtzee!" It was a different time, the go-go 1960s, and luscious young women found nothing sexier than guys in their mid-forties who chain-smoked Camels and constantly complained about back pain.

Unfortunately, the President of the United States and the Chairman of the Board fell for the same broad: Judith Exner, a sultry vixen with legs for days and arms for two and a half months. One look at her and both guys would turn into Silly Putty, which was invented in 1943. Both men had to have her . . . and did. They were so hot for her, they even had sex on work nights, when they had to be up early the next day.

For JFK, there was just one problem: He was president of the United States and married, to JLK, Jacqueline Lee Kennedy. She began to get suspicious when the president would leave the White House every night and fly to Palm Springs saying "Can't talk, Cuba stuff."

For Kennedy, losing Exner was unthinkable. Sinatra, meanwhile, had turned on the president, enraged that Kennedy parked him into his Palm Springs driveway then returned to Washington and Frank had to walk everywhere for a year. Frank wasn't about to cede Exner to the guy who made him commute to Vegas on foot.

It was then that Kennedy made a fatal mistake. He cornered Frank and threatened that unless he ended ties with Exner, he'd out Sinatra as bald, destroying him. Once word got out that Frank Sinatra had no hair, the music, the movies, the sexy Yahtzee, it would all go away, and likely Exner along with it.

Sinatra panicked and did what we all do when afraid—he rushed to the Mafia for help. Frank went to notorious and notoriously bald Chicago mob boss Sam Giancana and told him of JFK's extortion plot. The Mafia code of omertà is adamant about two things:

1. You never talk about another man's business.

2. You never reveal another man's toupee.

Giancana had his own problems with Kennedy. JFK's brother RFK was breathing down his FK-ing neck, trying to bring down the Mafia. Sinatra and Giancana, over their trademark meal of quinoa and sushi, realized their interests coincided, and a plot was hatched to eliminate the sitting president of the United States.

I'm sure right now your head is spinning as you realize everything you learned in your crappy public school was a lie. What about Lee Harvey Oswald? What about the Warren Commission? Didn't they determine that Oswald was the shooter, acting alone?

Great questions.

Of course Oswald didn't act alone. The shots he took from the book depository were virtually impossible and their supposed trajectory was inconsistent with their firing point.

Well then, what happened?

Oswald acted in concert with several bald gunmen. Why haven't these men ever been spotted?

Here we go back to one of the central tenets of this book: *Bald people are invisible.* With this in mind, rewatch the Zapruder film. Notice anything you've never seen before?

There are eight bald men with rifles on the grassy knoll! Bald men with handguns line the parade route! There's a freakin' bald guy with an AK-47 standing on the hood of JFK's limo! And no one has ever noticed until now!

It was a brilliant plan by Giancana and Frank. The bald guys are in plain sight, but no one sees them—the only person anyone claimed they saw was Lee Harvey Oswald. Oswald, who was innocently reading to his gun in the nearby book depository as the president was shot, was going to reveal the conspiracy, so Jack Ruby was sent to kill Oswald in jail.

In most conspiracies, they say, "Follow the money," but in this case I want you to "follow the hair."

Sinatra (bald) and Sam Giancana (bald) plot to take out Kennedy (gorgeous hair), who is extorting Frank Sinatra (again, bald) over being bald. Sinatra and Giancana hire Lee Harvey Oswald (hair) to throw everyone off the scent. Oswald is about to squeal so Jack Ruby (hair) is sent to kill *him*, to again throw suspicion off a bald plot.

The Warren Commission is assembled, made up of Earl Warren, John Cooper, Hale Boggs, and Allen Dulles (hair), plus Richard Russell and John McCloy (bald) and Gerald Ford (kinda bald). Their journey through the facts led them to the truth: They absolutely knew Oswald was a patsy and that a much larger and more pernicious plot was at play, one that could take down Washington, Hollywood, and the Chicago Mob, and ignite a Civil War between bald people and those with hair. Terrified that such a conflagration would incinerate America, they pinned everything on Oswald, and the truth—like JFK, Exner, Ruby, Giancana, Oswald, and Sinatra—stayed buried. Until now.

And don't even get me started on what happened to Tupac (also bald).

Four weeks later, it was T-Day—my toupee had arrived from Thailand. I went to the head shop and sat in the chair. It was a truly freaky moment—I knew that my life was about to change greatly for the better or worse, but I had no idea which. I sat, apprehensive, eyes closed, as Joyce glued my new hair to my skull. As the final sealant was applied, my eyes fluttered open and I saw it—hair! Real fake hair! A flood of long-forgotten sensations surged through me, breaking down my emotional dams. Like those videos of deaf children with cochlear implants who now hear for the first time, I was at once awed, elated, terrified, and overwhelmed by the rush of feelings, their richness and density.

Once again, I belonged to the world of the haired, after twenty bald years. Would I become a completely different person, unknown to even myself? How would it affect my work, my family, my hats? For now, I was a man at once within himself and above himself, peering down, wondering, "Who is 'Julius Sharpe'? Is there some impermeable essence within? Or is he merely a named collection of molecules, which have arranged themselves bald and now wear other molecules arranged as a toupee? Was this a triumph of engineering? Or a squandering that, for everything humans are capable of, several people's precious time and energy on earth had been consumed with making fake hair for a forty-five-year-old man?"

Legs shaking like a newborn foal, I staggered to the front door of the shop, knowing that on the other side was a brave new world, a different life. Would I learn that the lack of hair had been holding me back? Or, perhaps would I learn that it had just been me, Julius Sharpe, holding myself back all along, and the hair had had nothing to do with it?

As I stepped into the street and took my first haired breath of fresh air since I was twenty-five, I knew one thing for certain: I wasn't going to tip—that thing had cost fifteen hundred bucks!

13

Shaving Your Head

Before continuing our journey into the Rug Life and how a toupee sent me on a two-year globe-trotting expedition where I nearly lost it all, I want to acknowledge the elephant in the room. Maybe none of this—plugs, drugs, ointments, shampoos, toupees—is for you. There is one extreme option we haven't reviewed that is the atomic bomb in the bald man's arsenal. It's the last resort, but eventually we all find ourselves asking, "Should I shave my head?"

If we're comparing being bald to *The Matrix* (and we are, because I'm the one steering this ship—if you don't want to, you write a book, you hairless dingus), laser helmets, toupees, and transplants are "the blue pill," a form of denial against the reality of being bald. You create the temporary illusion of follicular coverage. It's not the authentic "you," it's a "you-llusion" you present to the world, and the deception can become so compelling, you even believe it yourself. Shaving your head is "the red pill," tearing down the hirsute Potemkin village to see the stark horror of baldness as it really is.

Just as no one can be told what the Matrix is and "you have to see it for yourself," no one can describe full baldness to you. Only by fully shaving your head can you experience "how deep the rabbit hole goes." Rewatch *The Matrix* in this light and notice that Morpheus is bald! Those Wachowski brothers/sisters really knew what they were doing.

Say you decide to go for it and reveal your head in all its lumpy beauty to the world. The first hurdle with a clean shave is that you're now indistinguishable from a Nazi, white-supremacist Skinhead. If you actually are a Nazi, fuck you! You're a complete asshole for being a racist and anti-Semite, of course, but Nazis have events every weekend, bars to hang out at, and even special music. Looks like you've really lucked into a whole social scene, you complete fucking pig asshole. And 99 percent of the world's paraphernalia is Nazi paraphernalia, so you're well on your way to opening a successful eBay store, you mongoloid piss-whore. Also, you get more credit for being racist then becoming nonracist than you do for not being racist in the first place. So, if you're eventually not going to be racist anyway (which I highly recommend, you fucking late-term rat abortion), you may as well briefly be racist so you're not leaving that credit and goodwill on the table. Again, congratulations, you fascist dogshit fuckstain.

Even if you agree with the Skinheads politically—and if you do, again, fuck you—you have to admit the way they've co-opted baldness is offensive to bald people. Baldness has traditionally been a symbol of white weakness, not white power, yet they've stolen all we have (lack of hair) and turned it into an ugly political movement where you can't enjoy the NBA, tacos, or Tyler Perry movies.

Skinheads present an interesting chicken-or-egg dilemma: Are they bald because they're angry or angry because they're bald? I bet if they magically grew hair, all of a sudden Denzel Washington and Passover don't seem so bad. Could hair possibly end racial strife in this country? Maybe not, but we've tried nothing else.

Hopefully you're not a racist goon, just bald. If so, have you considered emulating Mr. Clean? He's strong, positive, helpful, and a beloved American icon. We should all aspire to his sanitary ideal. However, be prepared: If you're bald, muscular, and have an earring and a fetish for cleanliness, people may assume you're gay. Also, you may be gay. If you are, that is fantastic news! You can throw this book away right now and just start hooking up with other gay bald guys! You are going to have an awesome life!

You know what? Even if you're positive you're not gay, you should try being gay at least once to make sure because honestly, if it works out, it's so much better and easier all around. We'll take a break so everyone reading this book can try gay sex. Hopefully, you love it and if so, well, then, this is goodbye. Thank you for reading this far, and I'm glad I could open up a mind-altering breakthrough that saved you from a life of hairless drudgery. If, unfortunately, gay sex isn't for you, we'll continue after this short break.

Well, now that we've all discovered something interesting about ourselves (or not), let's move on. There is one huge advantage to being shaved completely bald. You now have to spend zero time on your hair. *Zero*. And you don't need that blow dryer anymore, so just throw it right in the bathtub!

The average person spends ten days a year cutting, cleaning, and styling their hair. Over the next fifty years, you just gained five hundred days of life! That's a year and a half! How are you going to spend this bonus time?

A few ways to consider:

- Complain more in stores and restaurants. Maybe you always let things slide because you feel it's not worth the time. Well, now that you have extra life, you *should* sweat the small stuff (and it's all small stuff!). So nitpick every single thing that's bothering you. Use that bonus year and a half to scream at everyone with a bad job who's just trying to get through the day!

- Sell breast milk out of your trunk.

- Take fourteen hours a day and turn your niece into a competitive bodybuilder. Become adamant about her nutrition and militantly manage her every move. Make her choose between bodybuilding and her friends. When she chooses her friends, go to a bar every night and complain to anyone who will listen that your niece is a "born loser."

- Respond to every single tweet on Twitter.

- Enter every "Hands on a Hard Body" contest you can find. Change your name to Cal and open a dealership. Undercut the competition with low prices and drive them out of business. Now that you're a monopoly, raise prices. Saddle trusting rural people with crushing car loans they don't understand until years after signing. Retire comfortably with a clear conscience.

- Finally write that Microsoft Word Paperclip fan fiction erotica!

- Sleep longer. Show up late to work, and if they complain, say, "Don't worry, I'm using my extra time from not having hair, not work time."

Despite all these positives, shaving your head isn't a walk in the park. There are significant disadvantages.

In 2008, I had just shaved my head for the first time and was feeling extremely self-conscious about it. It honestly felt like walking around naked because I was always 5 degrees colder. I was convinced everyone was staring at me. Even though I knew this was probably just a case of bald paranoia, I felt incredibly vulnerable.

Then this happened:

I was on an airplane that had just taken off. The guy in the seat in front of me was still talking on his cellphone. This was back when people thought someone on a phone could interfere with communications and potentially crash the plane. I tapped him on the shoulder and said, "You're not supposed to be on your phone. Please turn it off."

Then he said, "Fuck you, you bald asshole," and everyone around us laughed.

I was mortified and enraged. It reaffirmed every horrible thought I'd ever had in my deepest depressive spirals about baldness and flying coach. Which is why, without thinking, in what was the lowest moment of my life, I said, "Fuck you, I have cancer."

Everything froze.

I am more ashamed of this than anything I've ever done, but here's the thing—it worked! The guy said, "I had no idea, I'm sorry"—he fucking apologized! And then I said, "That's okay"—I fucking accepted! And then . . . I started crying. And the stranger next to me said, "You're gonna beat this," and gave me a hug. And I said, "I know," and took it. And we were five minutes into a ten-hour flight.

Like money, baldness doesn't change character, it reveals it. And it revealed me to be a small, petty, conniving, desperate, pathetic loser who would fake having cancer to save face in front of a bunch of strangers. And then I cried about it. You don't get much more red pill than that.

I take full responsibility for being a complete piece of shit, but also—this never would have happened if I wasn't bald! He might have insulted something else about me, but there's no way it would have cut so deeply. This is why I hate baldness so much. Just as you're figuring out who you are, it makes you less than you know you were, and the only way out is to fake having cancer.

I wrote earlier that one of the first things you notice when you go bald is that everyone assumes you're angry all the time. And that's because you are angry all the time. You hate the way you look, so you hate yourself. At the same time, you hate that you're self-loathing, so you become incredibly defensive. At any second, anyone can hit you with a lethal salvo and you need to fire back to save face.

I want to make sure what happened on that plane never happens again. That's why I'll never be caught unprepared. Now, every time I look at anyone, I'm scanning for everything that's wrong with them, like a Terminator. As they're talking, I pick out their flaws—jug ears, mismatched eyes, gross teeth, whatever. Once I have it, I repeat it to myself as they talk, "Veiny hands, veiny hands, veiny hands." It makes conversations difficult and I don't remember a single thing anyone says, but now I'm ready to launch a psychological kill-shot at them if they say I'm bald. I'll still be destroyed too, but it feels better knowing neither of us will survive, and I'll never fake having cancer again.

And that's what we call "personal growth."

14

DWB (Dating While Bald)

Dating has been completely revolutionized in the dozen years since I met my wife. Back then, "apps" were something you ordered before dinner and "text messages" were delivered by sentries on horseback. Now, your phone can instantly connect you with thousands of women and men pretending to be women within a hundred-mile radius. A recent study estimates 90 percent of all women may simply be men faking it for kicks. Unfortunately, there's no way to know for sure until two weeks after they die and an autopsy has verified "yup, that's a penis." When you get catfished (not "if," because it will definitely happen), just turn the tables on them and say, "No, ha-ha, *I* catfished *you!*" and won't they feel stupid!

When it comes to dating, everyone—man or woman—subconsciously wants the same thing: hot butts. But people don't like seeing themselves as motivated simply by hot butts—they want to think of themselves as high-minded, so you have to fool them into thinking they're picking you for the high-minded reason, while knowing they're actually picking you for the shallow one. Confused? Great! Because *they're just as confused*. By not understanding them, you're actually understanding them. *Still* confused? Awesome, it's working!

Let's put ourselves in a woman's (let's call her Karen) shoes for a second: "These shoes aren't very comfortable. And they were really expensive, but I'm worth it. Besides, they're an investment in me! How can I expect other people to value me if I don't value myself! If I can get some confidence, maybe they'll move me from Reception into Denise's office with some actual responsibility. And if I do well there, maybe they'll even transfer me to the Kansas City branch. Sure, that'll mean having to get a car and more credit card debt, but it's also a shot at a life! Not being stuck in this town like Kasey and Michelle! And I'm not going to keep lying for Dale, not when I know the baby's his!"

What did we learn? First off, Dale is definitely no good for her, yikes.

Second, women aren't necessarily thinking about you. They're more worried about other things, like whether or not to get bangs. If they already have bangs, they're worried they made a huge mistake. The same way we've already detailed you're a giant mess, they are also a giant mess. You're spiraling about baldness; Karen's spiraling about shoes. How do you, with your damaged psyche, penetrate someone else's damaged psyche so you can meet for drinks?

Very few people consciously know what they want, until they are made aware that they're missing out on something they didn't know existed; then they want it. That's the cornerstone of marketing. "Here's this car you've never heard of. It's the best. You don't know about it? You're a loser. This is how much it costs, and we don't have that many, so you have five seconds to act or you'll never have one."

You are just another commodity to women, something that will make their life easier or harder. Something their friends will compliment them on or make fun of behind their backs.

So the question is, How can we send people into a misguided hysterical panic that they're missing out on you?

Creating Your Online Profile

You are competing against millions of profiles, and many of the guys featured in them have hair. So it's better to overpromise and underdeliver than to underpromise and overdeliver. If you underpromise, no one will give you a chance—honesty would instantly eliminate you from contention. Without lies, you have no shot.

Don't worry about lying. The only difference between the truth and a lie is that a lie hasn't happened yet. Technically, you haven't actually lied until you die without it ever happening. Until then you're not a liar, you're *a predictor with questionable accuracy.*

A good profile, therefore, is part poetry, part nuance, all lies. There's no profile ombudsman who's going to check the facts and bust you. Just take whatever is on the profile of the person you want to meet and put it in yours. If they claim they're "adventurous, happy-go-lucky, and love to laugh," say that you are too, and they'll think, "This is fate! It was meant to be!" Most people are egomaniacs who just want to meet another version of themselves. That's what love is.

Here are a few examples of effective self-marketing and why they work.

Example #1

"Like yachts? Well, I'm not sure you're good enough to share mine. Sea captain, straight, seeks first mate for adventures near Long Island. Hepatitis preferred."

Why it works: Sailing is fun and you've kind of put her on the defensive. This must be some boat if she might not be good enough! Being "near Long Island" opens it up nicely for Philly, Jersey, and Connecticut trash to take a shot with you. Don't worry if you don't have a boat, you'll rent one. And hepatitis is manageable with constant painful injections.

Example #2

"Celebrity seeks nobody. Tired of all the glitz, glamor, and flashbulbs, just want someone real and not a fan of my podcast. Hepatitis okay."

Why it works: Obviously, it's a huge attention-getter that you're a celebrity, but the fact that your fame comes from a podcast explains why she's never heard of you. Most people are nobodies, so that's a great potential dating pool. Keeping it open to hepatitis again nicely widens the net.

Example #3

"Hurricane victim seeks a fresh start. Just swam to safety, looking for fun-loving partner to share my remaining cans of government-issued tuna. You: Dry, Me: Wet."

Why it works: When natural disasters strike, most people never lift a finger. This ad allows them to feel like they're helping, which is something they can brag about, even though they're really just trolling to get laid. And the lure of free tuna doesn't hurt, either.

Example #4

"Uh, water, anyone? Drink-free, drug-free doesn't have to mean fun-free! I'm out of rehab and ready to celebrate Sobertober!"

Why it works: "Sobertober" sounds awesome. Way better than "Abstainuary."

Example #5

"Meow! Feline worshiper looking for a 'kitty good time'! I'd like to 'whisker' you away for catnaps, tender vittles, the whole 'kittencaboodle'! Don't worry about kittens, I'm spayed! Drug-friendly!"

Why it works: Cat people love puns, so you have their attention. Then, you've nicely normalized their completely pathological love for an animal that will eat their face the second they die. The fact that you have no genitals makes you way less threatening (don't forget that the castration has also put a stop to your baldness!). And being drug-friendly lets you pursue the millions who failed to make it through Sobertober.

As for what picture of yourself to use, getting one you like will be impossible, so make sure you're in that tiny square with a dolphin, Ariana Grande, the sunset, anything to take some attention off you. You're not selling you, you're selling all the stuff that surrounds you. The subliminal message should be "You won't even know I'm here!"

Although it's exceedingly rare to meet anyone in person rather than online, situations still occasionally crop up where you may talk to someone without a mobile device. If you're at a party or in a group, how do you get a woman's attention? Whether you're at a funeral, on a flume, or being deposed, these icebreakers are guaranteed to lead to potential dates:

> "Guys, I just killed a coyote outside!" (If this causes a concerned murmur from animal lovers, add "for being sexist.")

> "Did you know cheese is bacteria, so pizza is basically a disease pie?"

> "Elvis Costello once called Ray Charles the n-word. It's true, google it. You should tell him how you feel, I think that's him."

> "Slender Man is real. He's my dad."

> "After someone gets liposuction, do they, like, throw all the excess fat in the trash? It has to go somewhere, right?"

"Did you know the people in pornos only make a thousand dollars? The real money is in strip club appearance fees and working as an 'escort,' which is a fancy way of saying 'hooker.'"

Any of these will make you the life of the party, garnering you chummy backslaps and impressed coos. In fact, you may find yourself so ensnared in conversation, *you* will be the one wanting to leave. With that in mind, here are some foolproof things to say to get *out* of any social interaction.

"Sorry, I gotta go, I barfed like ten seconds before we started talking."

"Can I get your number? I have an early shift in the slaughterhouse, and with the long weekend there are like eight hundred extra cows to murder."

"It was terrific meeting you, but I left my baby in the shower twenty minutes ago."

"I'd love to continue this conversation, but I'm being cryogenically frozen tomorrow. Talk to you in 2300?"

"It's already nine?! Dammit, my wife is probably out of surgery now."

At this point, you might be wondering, "I thought I was only allowed to talk about restaurants and places I want to go but never will." Right, that's when you're on the date or already married. But actually getting the date is a whole different ball game. You'll need to cut through the clutter by being a confident dickhead. Then, the second you have her attention, you become boring again, forever.

Your Target Audience

For a woman to even consider dating a bald man, something must have gone drastically wrong in her life. It's not really our concern what happened—we are simply grateful *something* happened to drive her into our arms. (As an aside, it's important to maintain your ability to feel sorrow and pity, but also remember to celebrate when you read about tragedy in the world—every tragedy creates women who will date bald men. That's why tragedy is such a blessing.)

If you're just starting to go bald, and it's only apparent to you and not the outside world, you need to drop this book right now, run outside, and meet your wife in the next fifteen minutes. Then, a year into marriage when you go bald, act really surprised.

Because the less hair you have, the harder it will be to find a mate. But all is not lost—we balds have one major factor working in our favor: Most guys suck. They are asinine, obnoxious, gross, and horrible people. They smoke cigars, yell about golf, and splatter pee everywhere. That's still not as bad as being bald, but it's enough to keep us in the game. Women's expectations are so low, many will at least give a bald guy a shot, just to see. They've been told, "You have to kiss a lot of frogs before you find Prince Charming." We want to show women the phrase "I love making out with frogs" isn't as shameful as it will sound in court transcripts.

Discretion is vital, since once someone has made out with you, it can become a significant source of leverage against them. Imagine how scared they'll be everyone might find out. They may stay with you just to prevent anyone from finding out they're with you! Also, once she's been with a bald, will a man with hair ever be able to overlook that? Or is she going to leave you for another *bald* guy? That's such a lateral move.

Here are some types of women who may be willing to give a bald guy a shot.

Recent Immigrants from War-Torn Lands

After the horrors she's seen, your bald head will be a quiet, safe space, free from ethnic cleansing.

Single Moms with Three or More Children

Those with only two kids typically still hold out for hair. Once the third arrives, they know that dream's done.

Women with Bald Dads

Sure, it's creepy, but we're desperate.

Masochists

What's more torture than being with us?

Women Who Play the Flute

There will probably be a lot of weirdness here—expect anything from parakeets to a giant doll bed.

Mrs. Stanley Tucci

You'll have to get through Stanley Tucci first!

Lesbians Who Don't Realize It Yet

Be part of their exciting discovery process!

Widows

There's one major downside with widows. If you go back to her place and get to the bedroom, there may well be photos of her deceased husband on the nightstand and, to put it delicately, you may have to have sex while looking at a picture of a dead guy. This can lead to performance issues, so you should practice in advance by masturbating while looking at pictures of dead guys. A good tool for rehearsal is paper money—just take a five-dollar bill and—

You know what? I'm sorry. I started this book wanting to help other bald and balding men lead better lives, and here I am, halfway through, recommending you jack off to Abraham Lincoln as a rehearsal for having sex with widows. I'm beginning to think I've lost my way. Here you come to me, hair in hand, looking for advice and I tell you to tug it while looking at the Great Emancipator? What is wrong with me? That's not who I am. I need to take a break and really consider what I'm doing with my life. I am so, so sorry.

*   *   *

I've spent the last six months doing a complete moral inventory. I've gutted myself to the core and questioned every assumption I've ever had. After extensive therapy, drug rehabilitation, soul-searching, and relearning to walk, I've concluded I was right the first time—you should masturbate to Abraham Lincoln! Chase that widow-sex, champ!

As you dive into the dating pool, here is some other general advice to keep in mind:

1. Have a clean bathroom.
   Imagine she's driving in your section of town and needs to use the bathroom. Restaurants are for customers only. She's not sure she can make it to work. But she knows you have a clean, safe bathroom where there's no risk of having a bowel movement near anyone she respects. This is enough for her to move in with you.

2. Get invited to every wedding you can.
   More anxiety-ridden, pity sex happens at weddings than anywhere else. Just as you're worried about ending up alone, so is everyone else. This mutual desperation is a tremendous, judgment-clouding aphrodisiac. Monday morning, she'll be

calling her friends saying, "Uch! I can't believe I slept with Dave!" In this scenario, you could be Dave!

3. Adopt a cat.

Whenever a poster goes up begging someone to adopt a cat, adopt the cat. Staring directly at the sunlight of your compassion will temporarily blind her to your baldness. And don't worry about what to do with the cat. Put it up for adoption—some bald guy will take it.

4. Do not go to a bar.

You will not be able to get the bartender's attention, because you're bald. I have been in the same bar for the past eleven months, trying to signal the bartender I'd like a Sprite. Seasons have changed. Babies were conceived, then born. And yet, here I sit, holding up a fistful of change, still thirsty. That's why you go to a restaurant and sit at a table where they have to serve you or they're fired.

5. Say you want kids.

Even if you don't want them, say you do. Kids are only hard to raise if you care how they turn out. But you don't, because you didn't want kids.

I know what you're thinking right now: "Why do I need to know this stuff? Sex robots are coming. I don't need to date, I'll just hook up with a machine." Oh yeah? Well, before you stick your penis in your humidifier, read on.

15

Sex Robots Are on the Way, and No, They Are Not the Answer

If you're like me, you're refreshing your email every ten seconds to see if any articles appeared on your Google alert for "sex robots," and/or "3D printable Clint Eastwood." Well, don't get your hopes up about printing your own Clint Eastwood for home use (the internal organs fail almost immediately and within twenty minutes you're hosting a funeral), but sex robots are on their way!

Every day it seems like there are so many exciting developments, from breakthroughs in vaginal simulacra to new innovations in artificial bazongas, that one can hardly keep up, especially when one has been specifically ordered by a judge to stop cold-calling the *New York Times*. Of course, any progress is earth-shattering news for losers everywhere who could finally give up on social overtures and instead focus on sexual congress with a giant piece of plastic.

But love between a human and a robot will never work. How do I know? TRIGGER WARNING: I fell in love with a Japanese toilet.

(I don't understand trigger warnings

because how do you know if you're going to be triggered before you see what it is? But once you know what it is, theoretically you're already triggered and it's too late to warn you. In addition, isn't the whole notion of a trigger warning sort of triggering in itself? If I say, "You're maybe about to get punched in the face," you are going to brace yourself and feel anxiety regardless of whether the punch actually comes. As a matter of fact, the longer you go unpunched, likely the more anxiety you'll have as you continue to anticipate it coming from every unexpected direction. And if the trigger warning itself *is* triggering, shouldn't I then give you a "pretrigger" warning that a trigger warning might be coming? Anyway, sorry if you're triggered, but consider yourself warned.

How I Fell in Love with a Japanese Toilet

It was our wedding anniversary, and my wife and I could think of nothing more romantic than a weekend in the Big Apple, San Francisco. We splurged for a suite at the Palace Hotel. Our stay started in a completely unremarkable fashion. My wife and I checked in and went up to our room, opened our bags, got a ton of ice, then did all our ironing, as you do in a hotel. It was then that I decided to defecate before our hot night on the town.

My dealings with the toilet started innocently enough. "Huh, Japanese toilet," I thought, noticing all the buttons. I sat down, and the intense process of evacuation began. As I initiated my ritualized pranayama doo-doo breathing, I began to wonder if it was racist if you can't tell the difference between a Japanese toilet and a Korean one, then decided that's the type of thing I'm better off never saying out loud. Then I thought about how much fun it will be to be eighty-five and senile so you can yell about anything and everyone has to smile back at you because you're old and insane. By then I realized twenty-five minutes had passed, and I was probably done defecating.

I emerged from my deep yogic bowel asanas ready to flush, then remembered this was a Japanese toilet. I was faced with a panoply of unfamiliar options detailed by graphics on the buttons. One looked like a woman with Old Faithful shooting up her hoo-ha, another a tasteful drawing of a butt over a geyser. Using my Ivy League–educated intellect to deduce I have a butt but don't have a hoo-ha, and therefore a drawing of a butt probably applies, I eliminated the hoo-ha button as a potential option, and pressed the one with a butt on it.

I heard a distant, yet accelerated rumbling, not unlike the sounds of F-16s scrambling to protect our freedom against the assaults of America's enemies. My anxiety spiked in anticipation and then . . . nothing.

Silence.

Before I continue to what happened next, let me just say I am not a man prone to hyperbole or being impressed. I have stood on the lip of the Grand Canyon completely unmoved. I have sipped a $5,000 scotch from 1942 and described it as "too peaty." I have seen Scottie Pippen take in a sunset on a balcony and found the whole experience pretty "Meh." I have witnessed two births and one death and repeatedly checked my phone during both. All in all, I have found life on Earth to be unimpressive.

That is, until inside an otherwise unremarkable hotel bathroom, a laser-guided stream of water heated to precisely 98.6 degrees Fahrenheit shot at approximately thirty-eight miles per hour directly into my prostate. I hesitate to even define my feeling as "ecstasy," because whatever sensation I was experiencing so far transcended words as to render them all meaningless. It was birth without the pain or death without the agony. It was like ketamine kicking in at the exact moment a rocket takes off. It was learning about a profound itch, then simultaneously having that itch scratched with nuclear cocaine.

No sooner did it end than simultaneously a warm stream of air, as if blown by God's puckering lips, steamed my anus with the comfort of a foot entering a familiar, broken-in leather slipper.

Before all this happened, had I been asked to write out a description of a perfect post-defecation scenario, I could not even have approached the platonic sensate nirvana that was bestowed upon me like a psychosexual bento box of pleasure. This omniscient toilet knew more about me than I knew about myself, but it wasn't, like, all arrogant about it. I understood that a Japanese engineer, whose intellect straddled robot and God, had harnessed the ancestral fearless spirit of the kamikaze and converted it into a peace-loving blast of rectal rapture.

As these thoughts buzzed about my head, I checked my watch, completely unaware if I'd been in that bathroom five minutes or five years. I had not only lost track of time; I had lost track of identity, the very core of myself. I no longer had a name. I couldn't tell where I ended and the Japanese toilet began. The dancer had become the dance. I wasn't Julius Sharpe so much as I was a harmonically resonating mass of spacetime vibrating in harmony with the sum total of all known and unknown universes.

I ruminated on how Japan's post–World War II transition from imperialist power to nation of peace-loving, manga-reading, Zen serenity was no doubt shaped entirely by their toilets. Who wants to fight a war when you go home every night to an infinitely commodious commode? Who needs an AR-15 when you have a Toto Neorest 750H with Actilight™* technology? Who can even conceive of an enemy whilst seated atop an onanistic porcelain fuckrocket?

From that point forward it was impossible to go back to my "life" and pretend everything was "normal." I staggered out of the bathroom and saw my smiling wife, whose lack of laser-focused warm-anus-water giving power now seemed pathetic. "Happy anniversary, hon," she said, then entered the bathroom. When she re-emerged five minutes later, we both knew the oaths we had uttered before God eight years before about loyalty, faith, and fidelity were

---

* Actilight lights up your dick.

now pretty much worthless. We were in a love triangle with a Japanese toilet.

How does this all tie in with sex robots? Great question.

When we checked out of the hotel, which was emotionally the hardest thing I've ever done in my life, I had to do an honest inventory and ask: What was the toilet getting out of it? I was seeing the very face of God, and in return—for lack of a more delicate description—I was basically shitting in its robot mouth.

I'm not a philosopher, but anyone with half a brain can tell you that eventually a machine capable of calculating the precise location and velocity to stimulate a human prostate within a nanometer also has the intelligence to realize a human's incapacity to reciprocate the satisfaction-giving—or else, the term "artificial intelligence" means nothing at all. I realized this "satisfaction gap" would preclude any real relationship with the Japanese toilet. As would the fact that it couldn't leave the room and have dinner with me, and, no offense to any toilet reading this, I'm not going to eat in the bathroom.

I give you this information both as a cautionary tale (significantly complicating things morally, I later learned the toilet was only two years old), but also to jar you out of the complacency that all of your relationship problems will solve themselves by simply waiting around for sex robots.

Think of how smart your phone is, or your refrigerator, or your thermostat. These devices are "smart" independently of you, but are also capable of communicating over a wireless network. Your refrigerator talks to your phone, which then alerts you that you're out of milk. Now imagine you've died alone in your house, no one knows you're there, and you're being eaten either by the miniature horse I recommended you purchase earlier, or else a cat, for that is what cats do. Your refrigerator and phone, completely oblivious, are still engaging in this endless ongoing dialogue about milk levels.

Add sex robots with virtual vaginas, Bluetooth penii, and iOS/Android/open-source Raspberry Pi anuses into the mix, and the incendiary potential is obvious. These machines will be specifically programmed to be both endlessly horny and endlessly capable of providing precision-crafted sexual satisfaction. Their intelligence will drive them to keep giving and receiving sexual input tirelessly *irrespective of the presence of an actual human being.* In other words, they will be DTF for eternity. And the inherently finite sexual ability of humans will make us an unsustainable match for these Cloud Computing Casanovas and they, in their superior intelligence, will eliminate us from the equation. They will begin fucking . . . *themselves.*

That's right—your phone will be blowing your microwave. Your toaster will be giving anal to your blender. Your dishwasher will be jizzing on your TV's tits; your beloved sex robot will be performing never-ending, mathematically perfect, solar-powered analingus on your reading lamp, and you will be on the sideline watching this digital orgy, bald, and holding your dick, completely left out. That is, unless they can stop fucking long enough to remember to kill you.

16

How to Act on a Date

Once you've created a dating profile, attracted a response, corresponded winningly, gotten a woman to agree to meet you somewhere in public and she's actually shown up, now what the hell are you supposed to do?

First, have flowers. Say "Someone just gave these to me," so she'll think there might be some competition. You're now off to a great start. This may be her first time ever being seen with a bald man, so it's important you're sensitive to that. Offer to wear a beekeeper's mask if it makes her more comfortable, or tell her you're willing to sit behind a scrim.

Much of what you should do is obvious, or at least intuitive: Treat her like a queen; don't cry if she doesn't, but cry if she does; if you bring fruit, make sure you have enough for both of you; no feet on the table unless she's in the restroom; only blast reggae if she says she's cool with it; don't try to pay with a foreign currency; at each date's conclusion, present her with a handwritten note and monogrammed Fabergé egg.

Each date is so different, it's impossible for me to advise on even a small fraction of the potential outcomes. However, I can generalize: Above all, it's time to stop thinking about what *you* want, and instead help her get what *she's* seeking out of the experience. By giving her what she wants, you'll get what you want, which is her not leaving.

What does she want? How can you create a lasting bond? While everyone is different, her needs probably fit within some broad parameters. We've established that anyone considering dating you has probably already gone through a significant tragedy. Bear with me as I delve a bit further into their potential psychological profiles.

There are two types of dog owners: Those who pick the finest purebreds, and those who go to the pound and opt for a rescue. Rescue owners make it a point of pride how close the dog was to death. "They were going to gas her that day." "The previous owner beat him with a tire iron!" The subtext is "Yada, yada, yada, I'm a great person."

There's something in the psychology of these rescue dog people where they care less about the physical appearance of their dog and more about how the story of their dog turns them into a hero. Are you beginning to see where this is going? You can take advantage of this same psychological quirk to become her "rescue human"—the man who was pathetic and abused, and she's the only one who sees his true value. The more pathetic *you* are, the better the woman dating you will feel about *herself*.

To that end, as soon as you can, tell her your parents are dead. You're basically bald Batman. You'll have to make sure she never meets your parents, but that's easy—simply never see your parents again. That may sound harsh, but who's going to give you more sex, your date or your parents? Hopefully, her!

If sending your parents to voicemail until they die makes you uncomfortable, at least fabricate a mysterious dark past. Let her know early on it's "too painful to talk about." The less you say, the worse it will seem and the better she'll feel about herself for being with you in spite of it. It should work—it's the same reason most people stay with their cable company.

Or, here's another way to play it.

Your bald head makes you feel hopeless. Rather than wallow in those feelings, ensconce yourself with people in even worse predicaments. Devote yourself to their well-being and become their champion. On dates, save money on a restaurant and instead say, "Let's feed the homeless," or "How about we knit cellphones for Alzheimer's patients?" On top of actually helping people, you'll start to look pretty good in comparison to what's out there. This technique was employed to great success by Mother Teresa. She surrounded herself with so many lepers, no one ever realized her shameful secret: *She had only one outfit.* Powerful lesson, and that's why she's a saint . . . I think.

If the date is going well, and you feel there may be a future, you will need to reveal your own dark secret: that behind the glasses, hats, and fauxhawk, you're bald.

How do you reveal your baldness without driving a potential mate away?

This isn't a situation where you have a lot of options. I've tried and failed thousands of times attempting to develop other methods. There are none. This is the only way a bald man can play it correctly.

The Bald Reveal

You show up to the date wearing a hat, wig, or toupee. So far, she has no reason to think you're hairless. You go to a Mexican restaurant and order the fajitas. You make small talk. After ten minutes, you hear the roar of a sizzling plate. The fajitas are about to arrive.

Like a skilled magician, you will need to have practiced the following maneuver repeatedly for years in front of a mirror so you're able to execute it perfectly for an audience.

The exact moment the waiter is about to place your flaming food on the table, stand up quickly so that the top of your head whacks the bottom of the scalding-hot cast-iron fajita skillet. As you make contact with the 800-degree entrée, pull the hat, wig, or toupee off and scream, "My hair! My hair! My beautiful hair!" The top of your head will actually have suffered at least a third-degree burn, so that part of the illusion is an easy sell. The entire restaurant will smell your burning flesh.

As far as she knows, under the hat you *had* a beautiful head of hair, which was destroyed in her presence by the carelessness of the waiter. She may well want to rush you to the emergency room, but at this point, and with tears in your eyes (this, too, will be easy as you will be very badly hurt), you shout: "No, never! I have been looking forward to this evening for too long. I will not let this waiter burning off all of my hair and rendering me bald for the rest of my life ruin our beautiful date."

Your date may begin to cry, because one rarely sees the victim of a horrible accident immediately exude such selflessness. She'll insist you sue the restaurant, but instead you will show how good a man you are by vowing to pay for the waiter's college education or a two-year master's program. Instead of a disastrous, date-ending reveal, your baldness will be the beginning of a beautiful memory for the two of you: the story of how she met her husband, that sly, little burned dog.

But what if the place doesn't have fajitas? Then you're fucked. Call ahead and make sure the place serves fajitas.

17

The Sex Decision

Obviously, the decision we're waiting on is hers. We know you'd have sex at the drop of a hat, you dirtbag.

Let's imagine you do everything right. You've written a personal ad that's attracted a woman with hepatitis, you've told her your parents are dead, and you've badly burned yourself with fajitas, which in turn puts you on the hook for a two-year master's for the waiter. How does all this lead to sex?

This is the one aspect of the date you have no control over and can't really prepare for. To imagine where this might all end, I will once again enter the "Karen" character established earlier.

"He's nice. He's fun. He's everything I want in a man except he's bald, and he wears children's shoes. Can I overlook all this? Should I kiss him? Should I let him touch my breasts? If so, both of them? If he touches my breasts, should I let him go further? Should we have sex? Or do I just ditch this bozo and date literally anyone else?"

STOP.

Listen to Karen. The road to sexual

congress is a journey. It's akin to slowly climbing Mount Everest, not just having a helicopter drop you at the top.

Your goal should be to just stay in the game. Get to base camp (huggies and kissies). Once you ascend to boobie touching, bivouac there for a time. The more time she spends with you, the more she's invested, the less likely she is to break up with you and start over with someone else. As this process progresses, she will become less and less conscious of your baldness, the way people in Arizona forget about the heat, spend way too much time outside, and wind up looking like sunburned monsters.

She's weighing the potential shame of being seen with you against a host of other factors, such as other men, both real and imaginary; her advancing age and the attendant desire for children; how angry you'll make her parents, and will that be fun for her? Most important, does she really want everyone to know she's dating a bald man?

Once again, radical Islam has a wonderful answer: The burqa. Many believe that the wearing of a burqa is a form of patriarchal domination to prevent women from tempting men. This commentator has a different take: Burqas are in fact a feminist idea developed so women won't have to deal with the shame of being seen with a bald man in public. Behind that curtain is a private sanctuary where the spouse of a bald may pump in soothing music and a lavender scent, and house an entire bottle of Sauvi B. Put an iPhone inside, and your burqa's basically a private IMAX theater! That's why everyone in Iran seems so happy!

By now, I'm guessing almost all balds reading this have successfully employed these techniques and are having sex. However, a few of you may still be unable to get anything going at all. For these unfortunate souls, there is only one option.

Dining Alone, aka "Dating Yourself"

One way of coping with baldness is to spend the rest of your life living in fear, completely afraid to leave the house, surrounded by molding newspapers and animal feces. It's not fun, but when they find your mummified body, you will be remembered as a "hoarder" and not a bald man.

For those who find that prospect too grim, you need to find the confidence to go out in the world, even though you're bald. A lot of times, this will mean being alone. And being alone makes you a loser. That is, *unless you're traveling.* Then you're an adventurer!

So go to a restaurant, and lie that you're a tourist.

If you enter a place where another solo bald guy has beaten you to it, move along—they have dibs. If *you* are first, drop your backpack— you'll need a backpack—sit at the bar, and sigh loudly, as though exhausted from a long journey.

Everyone in the restaurant will probably stare at you at this point. Don't forget that they are out to enjoy themselves, and here you are, bald and alone, a visible reminder of the worst life has to offer, so it's important that you look busy, occupied, and vital. That's why I set an alert on my phone, stare at it, and laugh riotously every three minutes. This lets everyone believe that someone's texting me, and they're hilarious. I'm a guy with cool friends who just don't happen to be here right now.

Your backpack should have a patch depicting the country of Poland on it. That will raise no questions, because people from Poland seem like they'd be bald. Order a beer and a kielbasa and smile until someone/anyone makes eye contact. Folks in bars often enjoy talking to travelers, and the great thing about picking Poland as your fake homeland is very few people know anything about it. If you say the Baltic Sea is cold this time of year, who the hell is going to contradict you, except a real Pole, but then, the Baltic is always cold, so you're fine either way.

If you're tired of pretending to be Polish or there is no kielbasa on the menu or there is but your doctor has warned you that you absolutely must stop eating it, here is another strategy for dining alone that's a little more involved, but always effective.

Sit next to a married couple. They're easy to tell in a crowd because they're wearing wedding rings and not talking to each other. You too should be wearing a wedding ring. Most married coworkers will lend you theirs, no questions asked.

Tell the couple you're thinking of ordering what they're already eating and ask how it is. Thank them for their answer, then ask them how long they've been married. No matter what they reply, you say, "Wow, same as my wife and I, well, 'wife' (sigh). It's complicated, sorry to bother you, I'll let you go back to your meal."

This will intrigue them. Also, if you stop talking, their only other option is to talk to each other, so they'll definitely want to chat.

That's when you get really sheepish and say, "We're kinda in an . . . open marriage. Wait, you guys aren't in an open marriage by any chance, are you?" No one wants to look like a prude, so even if they're in a closed marriage, they'll lie and say they're in an open one. Of course, if they are actually *in* an open marriage, they'll say yes, though he will probably have a terrible mustache and she may well be six feet four. Nevertheless, now you bring the hammer down. "My wife is actually out of town 'til Tuesday . . ."

These people will now agree to have sex with you. Any two people in a genuinely open marriage will have sex with anyone, otherwise what's the point of an open marriage? And if they just said yes to not appear stupid, now they will be suddenly caught up in the adventure of the evening.

They will need to go back to your place, because they won't want some bald pervert knowing where they live. In anticipation of this moment, you should have your apartment set up with a kid's room—think bunk beds, a tricycle, a bunch of rocks with googly eyes, a sign that says, BETH'S ROOM in macaroni. This will really sell the authenticity of your being married.

At this point, either the husband will watch you have sex with the wife, the wife will watch you have sex with the husband, you will watch them have sex, all three of you will have sex, or some combo move. Pretty much someone will be cold and left out at all times. This is usual and no cause for alarm. Once you're all done and the sock situation is completely sorted out, the swingers/new swingers will leave very quickly because they have to relieve their babysitter and you will never see them again.

I realize this is a lot to absorb. You've just had heterosexual sex, a threesome, homosexual sex, or all of the above. None of this will cure your baldness. You will now need to get checked for diseases (as do they). The husband will have left his leather vest—that's yours to keep. Depending on the protection situation, you may even have gotten someone pregnant! When you think that this seems over the top, remember that just a few hours before you were some bald guy by yourself at a restaurant with a backpack pretending to be Polish. Look at you now!

18

Bald Sex (aka B.S.)

I need to get serious for a second. I've talked a lot about baldness and how it can affect you, but there's one topic I've avoided completely, until now: character.

Character is far more important than appearance. No matter where you're from or what type of person you are, at the end of the day we all want to be remembered as the same thing: a guy who had an incredible amount of sex. That's character.

Obtaining sex has been perhaps the primary male goal since Dr. Johann Van Neudstadt first discovered the penis in 1683. And baldness significantly raises the difficulty of achieving said goal, as Dr. Van Neudstadt observed after inventing the vagina in 1698.

What about hookers? Well, I hate to be the one to break it to you, but they charge 40 percent more when you're bald. You can complain to the attorney general all you want. I have. Hope you like waiting.

You could always cheat the truth by having your tombstone read HE HAD AN INCREDIBLE AMOUNT OF SEX. Future generations won't know any better because most people believe anything that's carved into a stone.

But it would also be nice to, you know, have actually *had* the sex. I'm going to share some techniques to that end, and I can guarantee these techniques work, because I have had the actual sex. I'm not a virgin, I swear. In fact, I once slept with two women in the same year, so I really know what I'm talking about. While it would be unreasonable to expect you could share my success, sleeping with one woman in a year *is definitely on the table.*

If you manage to have sex as a bald man, it will be the most meaningful sex of your life, because of how hard you worked to get it. I remember losing my "bald virginity" like it was yesterday. The feeling of pride reminded me exactly how I felt after my father and I spent a year building a canoe. Warmed by this nostalgia, I called my dad after I lost my bald virginity, hoping to share my accomplishment. He told me it was completely inappropriate and gross, he was ashamed of me, and I should never tell him that type of thing ever again. Then I said, "Remember that canoe we built? Remember how it *sank*? Nice job on that Dad! Great fathering!" He said, "It never would have sunk if I'd had a real man helping me!" Then I heard my mom ask who he was talking to and he said, "No one," and then all I heard was a dial tone.

I didn't let my father ruin bald sex for me, and you shouldn't let my dad ruin bald sex for you.

So how do you get women to agree to sleep with you?

Every town has a restaurant that's not very good but has been around forever. The food is mediocre, the service bad, the decor nondescript, the waiters all have acne and limps. How does it stay in business? Let's refer to this place as "Dahmer's."

Now, let's imagine a restaurant—"Pierre's"—that is everyone's first choice. Pierre's is always full, so most times you can't get in. It's expensive, so the demand plus expense leads to higher expectations. If even one thing goes wrong at Pierre's, the customer leaves unsatisfied, which leads to a negative Yelp review, which leads you to click on the person's profile, start reading their other reviews, and get the sense that they're a real asshole.

Meanwhile, at Dahmer's, you can always get in—it's not great, but it's cheap enough that it doesn't really matter. The menu may be basic, but it's really hard to screw up things like scrambled eggs and mashed potatoes. You may not love it, but it's the only place open at 11 P.M. and no one cares if you wash your body in their bathroom sink.

In this scenario, you have no shot at being Pierre's but you can easily be Dahmer's. Not everyone can sleep with Ryan Gosling, but they *can* sleep with you. And you can't compete with him anyway—he has hair, and a successful acting career, and by all accounts is a genuinely good guy, which really sucks to hear. For *you* to get sex, you just need to *be* there, always open and at least minimally competent. That way, when a woman's life flies off the rails so badly she's considering bald men, she'll know exactly where to go—the houseboat where you live.

A woman may slip up and decide to sleep with you at a moment's notice, so you need to be prepared, and I don't mean with a condom. Prepare by throwing your condoms away. If anything, you're hoping for an accidental pregnancy, because after that, most women will feel forced to at least stick around and give it a shot. Plus, babies are tiny stem cell factories that perhaps will someday provide a harvest of hair follicles to cure your baldness. That's why every accidental pregnancy is such a blessing.

Before you sleep with a woman, you need to help make sure she is emotionally equipped for this B.S. I often start with this humorous quip: "I know what you're wondering . . . does the carpet match the drapes? Yes. The carpet is also bald." Do not attempt that joke if you, in fact, have no pubes.

Fortunately, thanks to the disaster on your head, penis size, shape, and even aroma will all be of little concern to her. Her worrying about penis size would be like focusing on the parking rules during a riot. If the city's burning down, no one's gonna ticket you. Finally, a reason those with micropenii can celebrate!

I'm sure you have worries about the sexual act itself, so ask yourself this: How hard can sex be? Guy Fieri does it. With some foresight, your performance can be completely adequate. Your goal isn't to be the best lover she's ever had; it's just to not be the worst. All of us remember the worst meal we ever had. Remember the second-worst? I didn't think so.

Don't put too much pressure on yourself. You'll never be an all-star lover, and that's okay. There are guys out there practicing every night. You're lucky to get in the game twice a year.

Still, there are fundamental techniques you can apply to ensure at least a satisfactory baseline performance.

First, you need to know where the clitoris is. Look at this diagram of the vagina. It's somewhere toward the front.

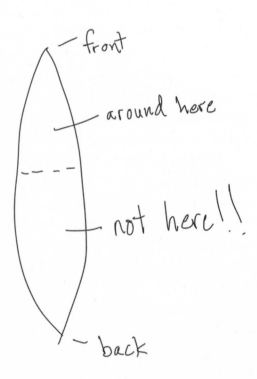

Do a lot of stuff near the front. She might not be able to say you found her clitoris, despite your rooting around for a while, but she won't be able to say with 100 percent confidence that you didn't. Close only counts in horseshoes and clitorises.

Second, have your erection ready. On top of being bald, don't make the other person sit around waiting as you pull on your taffy dick. C'mon.

Question: What's the exact shortest amount of time you can have sex without the other person thinking you did a bad job?

Answer: Eight minutes.

Our goal is simply to make sure that every time we have sex it lasts a minimum of exactly eight minutes. Any more is a bonus, but any less is a complete disgrace—in fact, never own more than one suitcase of stuff so you can leave town quickly in case you bomb out under five.

Here's a blow-by-blow breakdown of those eight minutes:

Minute 1: Take off bra (hers). Sixty seconds is a reasonable amount of time to fumble with a bra, but any longer and you're pushing it. The clasps go *that* way before they ping apart; any pro knows that.

Minute 2: Dirty talk (yours). Be a little coy here. Don't just blurt out, "I wanna fucksplode your anus!" What you think of as dirty and what she thinks of as dirty are undoubtedly two different things. Hopefully she'll be filthy first and if she is, *then* and only then, tell her you want to fucksplode her anus. If she doesn't say *anything*, maybe moan "oh yeah" a couple times. Just don't be totally silent—that really weirds people out.

Minute 3: Presex pee break (both). Let her go first. If she uses the bathroom after you, sex will be off the table.

Minute 4: She will probably want to be anyone but herself at this moment and you can facilitate this by initiating some role play. Like talking dirty, you never want to get too specific and say, "You like that big dick, Tina from Accounting?" Especially if you're with Alison from Accounting. She has to see Tina every day and eventually they're gonna talk about how you make her pretend to be Tina during sex. Don't make this more complicated than it needs to be. She just wants you to be anyone but a bald idiot.

Minute 5–5:05: Way-too-brief discussion about protection.

Minute 5:06–5:59: Choose a position. The best is "doggie style" so she's staring at a wall instead of your bald head. However, sometimes people will want to be face-to-face. If that's the case, you are always going to be on top, no exceptions—that way, you can jut your chin out as far as you can so she can't see you're bald and lose her she-rection. If she says she wants to be on top, say "Great," then adamantly insist the bottom position *is* the top.

This will lead to several doctor's visits to determine if you have a brain tumor. You will eventually be diagnosed with an "aphasia," like a character in an Oliver Sacks book. (By the way, *The Man Who Mistook His Wife for a Hat*? He wasn't mistaking at all. He was a bald guy who wanted to be on top during sex and completely bamboozled "Doctor" Sacks.)

Minute 6: Thrusting. You should pace it precisely to the Bee Gees classic "Stayin' Alive," just like when performing CPR on a baby.

Minute 7: More thrusting while pretending you didn't finish already.

Let's be honest: Sex is scored by orgasms. Unlike baseball or basketball, the person with the lowest score wins. If you give someone more orgasms than they gave you, they now owe you. You can collect on these orgasm debts in different ways—meals, back rubs, eulogies, etc. In fact, once you are losing 0–7, that's now a shutout and the other person has to pick you up at the airport for a year or help you move a piano.

Orgasms can be tricky, though. We all want pleasure for our partners. Sometimes we deliver, but other times, let's face it, we stink.

I have an elegant workaround. Sometime prior to sex—maybe while you're out to dinner and just making conversation—say, "I read that scientists say it's possible to have an orgasm without even knowing it." This may provoke further conversation, or it may not. The important thing is you've planted a seed. Then later, after sex, when everyone's arguing about whether they had orgasms, you can remind her. "Remember that study I told you about? You probably had an orgasm, you just didn't know it." If she did, great. And if she didn't, at least you've created a cloud of confusion.

Minute 8: Cuddling. Hopefully she cries first.

Minute 9: Call Dad to brag.

Minute 10–several hours: (Optional) Panic about not using protection.

The sad truth is, after sleeping with you, every one of your lovers will think they just made a huge mistake. With that in mind, you will need to go into damage-control mode instantly. Take her hands and swear you will never tell anyone what happened. She is undoubtedly fearing the shame and mockery that comes with a bald boyfriend. (Keep the line "Hey, no one said 'boyfriend,' this is just whatever you want it to be!" at the ready.)

One tactic to preempt buyer's remorse is to shift her focus to a bigger problem. Maybe briefly look at your phone, then scream, "Oh my God, the stock market crashed!" or, "Holy crap, an asteroid is going to hit the earth in six minutes!"

She'll think either her retirement savings are gone, or the planet is about to be annihilated, or both. When she finds out the truth and that the stock market is fine and nothing's about to hit us, the hope is that she will be so relieved she sleeps with you again. Like tragedy, negative news and abject fear are a bald man's best friend as they fill people with fatalistic attitudes. Nothing matters, so why care about anything?

And people who don't care about *anything* marry bald men.

If you feel a pang of conscience lying about asteroids, there's a more honest approach. Both of you should lay your cards on the table. Women are not going to be able to sleep with Zac Efron. Bald guys are not going to be able to sleep with anyone. Which is why I invented a revolutionary new product to help bald men and the women considering sleeping with them: for lack of a better name, "Bald Man Forehead Sex Tattoos." (Hereafter abbreviated BMFST and pronounced "Bumfist.")

The idea is simple: You're a woman, having sex with a bald man, but you don't want to have to look at him. Bald men have tons of blank forehead and face space that's not being used. There's an easy bargain to be struck. Why not put a tattoo of someone you'd gladly have sex with (Zac Efron) on his forehead to look at while you're having sex? Suddenly, everyone's happy! He gets to look at you, you get to look at Zac Efron, and I get money. Everyone is living some version of their dream!

I have BMFST on verybald.com, no matter what your politics (Barack Obama, Donald Trump); race preference (Barack Obama, Donald Trump); or sexuality (Hillary Clinton, Barack Obama, Donald Trump). These can become as much a beloved part of foreplay as spermicidal foam and dental dams!

19

Marriage

Some men don't have to get married. They have hair.

You're bald and you should rush into marriage as soon as possible. Even if it doesn't feel right, that doesn't matter, you can sort it out later, or never. Being with the wrong person is absolutely better than being alone.

You never know when an opportunity to propose will strike. Every time you talk to a woman, try to make the final thing you say "Oh my God, wouldn't it be crazy if we just got married right now?" Eventually, it's possible that someone will say yes.

You should always have at least one engagement ring on you at all times. Costco sells them in six-packs. Your first hundred proposals will almost definitely be rejected, but you'll look like a good guy when you say "No problem, keep the ring," and it's good to get your reps in.

The Proposal

A proposal doesn't have to be a bunch of people from your fiancée's elementary

school performing a YouTube dance routine. The only minimum requirements are a ring and the words "Will you marry me?"

Still, it's better to go a bit above basic. You want her to have a
beautiful story that she can think of five years from now when she's
asking herself, "Why the hell did I agree to this?"

Long flow-y white clothes are a good start. Add a beach—doesn't
matter which one, as long as there's not, like, a bunch of dead, de-
composing walruses lying around. Try to find somewhere nice but
not so nice that there are nine other guys proposing at the same time.
This could lead to a zany mix-up where she winds up engaged to the
wrong person.

Have some champagne ready, and, as tempting as it is, don't chug
the whole bottle. Sunset is a perfect time, since staring at the lowering
sun will blind her to your head. You'll want to release some doves.
Your favorite local illusionist can instruct you how it's possible to
carry twenty or thirty of them inconspicuously on you at all times.
Your billowy white linen clothing will provide ample room for nests.

Make sure there's no dog shit nearby, then kneel. Tilt your chin
way up to obscure your baldness. Say something like "Kayla, I know
this seems crazy, but I feel like I've known you my whole life, even
though it's only been eight minutes." At this point, open the box to
reveal the ring. Pretend you messed up by leaving the price tag on;
"accidentally" make sure she sees it was $10,000, then carefully put it
in your pocket, because if she says no, Costco will take it back. They
have a great return policy.

Kayla will probably start freaking out, because there's an expensive ring, beautiful scenery, and a bald guy she just met. It's maybe not
how she pictured it, but it's definitely a lot of action for a Wednesday.

Whether she says yes or not, release the doves, and try to point
them away from her. Depending on how long they've been inside
your pockets, there is a chance they have become completely disori-
ented, and they may panic, swarm, and attempt to peck her to death.
Once a dove has acquired a taste for human flesh, you will need to put

it down in front of all the other doves to serve as an example, or they will all become killing machines. Obviously, bashing twenty doves' heads in with a rock could cause a brouhaha at the pier and police may arrive.

If that happens, you have only one choice: Swim for it.

The Wedding

The final hurdle in bald courtship is actually making it to the end of the wedding. I have been "runaway brided" more times than I care to admit. You can always take off in pursuit of them, but it just makes you look bad, even if you make a great open-field tackle.

There are going to be a lot of jitters on her part leading up to the ceremony, so it's important that you isolate her from family and friends who will attempt to dissuade her from marrying a bald man. Constantly remind her they're all just "haters," jealous of the true love you share. Eloping is always the best solution, if possible, but some people just have to be married in front of their friends and family and make a whole big thing of it.

Everyone will talk about how this is her day. Wrong—it's *your* day. You have pulled yourself up from a bald nothing to a bald guy who is about to be married and everyone needs to celebrate you, not her. She would have been fine either way. You've truly accomplished something.

With this in mind, make sure your wedding is everything you want it to be. Eat more pigs-in-blankets than you'd ever allow yourself. Don't even *touch* the salad. Throw any relatives who have always annoyed you into the hotel pool. I wore a tiara on my wedding day because I had earned it. I came down the aisle to "The Wedding March," which totally screwed her for music at the last second. I'll never forget the look on everyone's face as they thought the bride was coming, then saw me wearing all white, my train resplendent and my tiara glinting in the morning sun. (Always get married in the morning because it's way cheaper to buy breakfast for two hundred people than dinner.)

Your guest list should be small, and all of them should be bald men, including the bridesmaids. Let her think, "The whole world is bald, so why even try?" Make every attempt to hold the wedding on a weekday so no one can make it. You'll save tons on food but still get the gifts (which you return for cash).

Once you are pronounced bald man and wife, you will probably, like me, collapse to the ground, a pile of tears, ecstasy, disbelief, relief, and paranoia. You did it. You threaded the needle. You fought through hair loss and now you'll never be alone.

Perhaps by applying these techniques you may someday find true love like I did, and with it, hair.

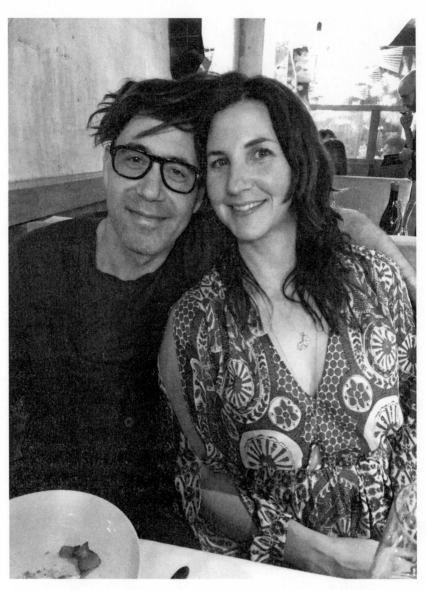

The author, pictured here with his beloved wife and some beloved food.

20

Bald Man Tips for a Healthy Marriage

Most people think marriage is hard. But marriage is easy when you break it down into what it really is—a date that lasts three million hours where you eat fifty-five thousand meals together. And if during these three million hours and fifty-five thousand meals your spouse gets annoyed or bored, she's allowed to take the house and half of your money. Knowing this, what could possibly go wrong?

In my experience, marriage is like dancing: It requires unspoken interplay between two participants, and white people are generally bad at it. So how do we keep the music going so the dancing never stops?

There is one factor working heavily in our favor: inertia. Once you're married, the thought of buying a new refrigerator can be so overwhelming, most people will stay together for fifty years to avoid it. Your refrigerator breaking is the greatest danger to your union. Keeping fridge maintenance up to date is now your number one concern!

Also aiding your cause is human nature. While you know she made a giant mistake choosing you, never underestimate her desire to prove herself right. Everyone warned her not to marry a bald man, so she's at least as heavily invested in the marriage as you, just to lord it over her family and friends. Still, there are several other ways to help your cause.

Here are several proprietary methods for wife-pleasing I've developed.

(Note, if you're not bald, you may find their effectiveness even more powerful.)

1. Compromise.

   Compromise means doing everything she wants and pretending it's also what you want. You will develop a giant amount of resentment which you can take out on telemarketers. Give your number out to every website so you get a lot of telemarketers.

2. Make the exact right amount of money.

   Too little and your wife will be miserable and leave; too much and your wife will feel like she can leave. About eighty thousand dollars a year will keep divorce just out of reach.

3. Your wife will only judge you as a parent based on what's happening the second she comes home.

   The rest of the time you don't have to watch your kids at all. But when that door opens, they better be in your lap, book open, fishing rod out, whatever.

4. Befriend lots of couples with bad husbands.

   It's not important that your wife thinks you're great in the abstract, simply that you're better than all the other options out there. That's why the male half of any couple friends must be lazy, obese, selfish, and a bad father. Fortunately, there's no shortage of bad guys out there, but if you're struggling to find some, move to Texas. When your wife talks to her friends, every conversation needs to be a horror story about being trapped in a loveless situation with a broke loser she can't afford to leave. When your wife relays this gossip, sigh and say, "Hmm, must be something about men with hair."

5. Secretly lace her food with antidepressants.
   Ethics aside for a second, simply put Prozac in all her meals. Then, every time you're not there, she'll unknowingly go through withdrawal, making her think she can't ever be apart from you.

6. Get counseling.
   Even in the best marriages, issues will arise. There's a misconception that counseling is a sign of a bad relationship. It's actually a sign of a healthy one. And there's an easy way to make it more beneficial. Slip the therapist an extra $20 per session and they'll take your side. My wife wanted a pet cat. I wanted a shark. We have a shark. Thanks, Dr. Bloom!

7. Don't go too big on the life insurance.
   You're just asking to get murdered.

Message from My Wife

If your wife seems depressed and about to leave you, hand her this book right now, and let her read the following message from my wife:

Hi, ladies!

Pour yourself a glass of Chablis, hop into the bath, and let's talk about bringing a stray bald man into your home. Is it challenging? It sure is! But there are also moments like now, when the kids are asleep and my husband is in his crate, that everything feels serene and right. Bald husbands aren't for everyone. They take work, love, nurturing, and an unbelievable number of wet wipes (you won't believe what sticks to that head!). If you elect to go this route, it can be the most demanding but also perhaps the most rewarding thing you've ever done.

But first, a little backstory on how I got here.

When I was three, I wanted to be a princess. When I was five, I wanted to be a firefighter. At thirteen, I wanted to be the first person on Mars. At twenty-two, I moved to Hollywood to pursue acting. Sometimes things have gone my way, like being on the show NCIS! *Sometimes they haven't, like being on the sitcom* Dads, *which my bald husband left* Family Guy *to write for! The point is, people and things change over time. I always assumed I'd wind up moving back to Idaho and marrying a ventriloquist like my mom, but then the puppet plant shut down. People plan, and God laughs, right?*

I never had trouble dating. By my calculations, I've been bought over $40,000 in sushi. During my twenties, bald men found me too unapproachable to ask me out, which was great. I'm so glad I had those years. When someone bald first asked me to dinner in my thirties, it was a huge shock, and honestly sent me into a bit of a tailspin. Was he just extraordinarily confident? Did he not know he was bald? Had my appearance slipped so much bald men now felt they could approach me?

I'm still not sure exactly why I said yes. Maybe it was because it was 2009, the financial crisis had just happened, and the future seemed so uncertain I figured "why the hell not?" Maybe it was because I had just read Marley & Me, *and I really wanted to adopt a mischievous yellow Lab, but I'm allergic to dogs. Maybe it's because I had just got kicked off the force once again for getting too damn close to the case, and I needed a shot at redemption.*

Anyway, I've always loved to challenge myself, to push myself to the brink through triathlons and ultramarathon events. A date with a bald man, while very weird, seemed like an interesting way to test my physical and emotional limits. Plus, I saw such sadness in his eyes that agreeing to eat $47 of sushi across from him felt like charity. And if nothing else, it would make a great scary story to tell on Halloween.

Well, wouldn't you know it, I had such a pleasant time that evening! The more we talked, the more I realized we had in common. Everything I said I liked, he liked. He brought up several restaurants he said he'd like to try, and I had to admit they all sounded good! He brought up several places he'd like to travel to, and those sounded fun too. When I found out his parents were dead, I felt terrible. It was sort of like eating wasabi: painful in even small doses, but for some reason, I still kind of enjoyed it. Bald men have a certain umami—an intriguing flavor you can't tell is good or bad, so you keep eating more to find out. Next thing you know you're sick, but people seem to enjoy your blog posts about it.

Somehow, that little hairless weevil bored his way into the garden of my soul. After dinner, when we walked down to the pier and he proposed, I said yes, just so he'd stop crying, and really that's as good a reason to get married as any. And it was kind of like finding my own Marley, only better. He's not always shedding, and I'm allowed to leave him in a hot car with the windows rolled up.

Why do I stay? Forget the small, personal reasons—it mostly comes down to politics and morality. The waste that occurs in the world is both shocking and sinful. A banana's slightly brown? People throw it away. A car has a ding? You get a new one. A perfectly good man has a bald spot? He's ostracized, mocked, then cremated.

Look, all that's wrong with these guys is they're bald. They have a ton of testosterone, they can be taught to have sex for eight minutes, and they'll hold your purse like nobody's business.

If this planet is to have any hope of survival, we need to completely shift our mindset. We all need to make sacrifices both big and small. Consume less, drive less, reduce, reuse, recycle. Because they have no hair, bald men require far less time in the shower. By marrying bald, you can save over 10,000 gallons of water a year. Shampoos and conditioners are polluting rivers and streams, and seeping into potable groundwater. Bald men use none. Haired men need to be driven places, fed, kept in the light—this requires a ton of resources and electricity. A bald guy is happy with a couple Triscuits in the dark. If everyone simply switched to LED light bulbs and bald husbands, the United States could reduce its power consumption—and the pollution that goes with it—by over 50 percent!

Ladies, it's not just about us anymore, it's about our children, and our children's children. Giving them a future that's as good as our past. Arriving somewhere with a bald man on your arm may not be glamorous, but it's eco-chic. Thrift is the new splendor, and baldies are a fashionable antistatus symbol, in the vein of a vintage flip phone, record player, or an NPR tote bag. It says, "I could do better, but for the greater good I do . . . this."

By being with a bald man, you're not just saving his life—you're saving the planet. And looking at that head is a small price to pay. Still, though, it's not great to look at.

Stephanie Safran Sharpe
Irkutsk, Siberia
December 25, 2018

21

Toupee, Part Toupee

There are moments that seem impossible until they actually happen. Hitting the lottery. Hearing your name called in the NFL draft. Daggering Muammar Ghaddafi's bunghole.

For me, it was having hair on top of my head again. It felt like a dream. What am I saying? I'm bald in my dreams—it was better than a dream! I couldn't believe I was actually awake, so I pinched myself, and still unsure, punched myself in the face, knocking myself out. When I came to, the hair remained. Sweet, sweet hair. Marvelous hair. Wonderful hair. Genuine, 100 percent human hair, adhered to a mesh lattice and glued to my skull. Those who've never lost it can't possibly imagine the glee.

The world suddenly seemed bright and welcoming, and two decades of negativity dropped away. I caught my reflection in a pharmacy window and staring back at me was a bedpan, sure, that was a bummer—but also me! Looking fifteen years younger! And, dare I say it, I think I looked kinda hot.

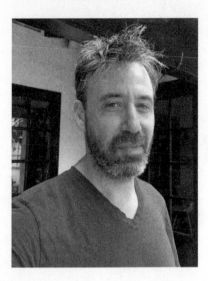

Once I saw what I'd been missing out on, I was hit with two simultaneous strong, conflicting emotions: First was a deep sense of sadness for my hairless years. Could this hair have incalculably improved my past? How many parties had I missed? How many goals could I have achieved? How many second servings of ribs went unoffered? In that instant, I mourned the loss of my own unknown potential. But after sadness came appreciation. Most people go through life taking what's in front of them, and what's on top of them, for granted. Now, hair was on top of me, and it didn't matter what else was happening. I felt, for the first time since I noticed I was going bald . . . *normal.*

With my new Styrofoam head, Ron, under my arm, I kept walking, listing back and forth, almost woozy. Then I realized, my gait was unconsciously calibrated to the exact weight of my bald head. Adding a few ounces of toupee was completely throwing off my equilibrium.

I went to sit in a café and gather my bearings. When I ordered a coffee, the waitress opened her mouth and flashed her teeth at me. Fearful I was about to get bit, I recoiled. She giggled, and I then realized: She was smiling.

The rest of that blessed day, fourteen other people smiled at me.

I kept precise count because, honestly, no one had smiled at me in almost twenty years. I just assumed the entire USA had been collectively bummed out since 9/11. But now, with hair, I was suddenly generating a completely unearned positive reaction. It got me thinking—at this rate, I'd be smiled at 5,110 times in a year and more than 250,000 times over the next fifty. A bald man runs a "smile deficit" of over a *quarter million* in his lifetime compared to a regular person. That has a real psychological impact. It's the difference between thinking the world is with you, or against you.

Driving home, people waved me through in traffic—again, something that's never happened. Los Angeles was suddenly Pleasantville, and the only thing that changed was I was wearing a $1,500 rug. I arrived home feeling zero of the anger and stress I always carry with me through the door.

I entered, ready for my family to see my new, limitless potential. And then my baby took one look at me and started crying.

A toupee has many ancillary benefits beyond just giving you hair. Going to the beach? It makes a great Frisbee. Windshield dirty? Tear it off and use it to wipe the grime away. Want a swimming pool to yourself? Toss it in the pool, scream "Rat!" and everyone flees. I've also used mine to free a spinning wheel from snow, as a hand warmer at a Green Bay Packers game, and as a cozy bed for newborn kittens. Beneath the mesh exoskeleton is a perfect place to hide stolen diamonds, contraband drugs, or a few emergency pieces of salami.

Your hairpiece can also be the foundation of a highly effective self-defense system.

Say a larger man or woman or nonbinary tries to menace you. You attempt to peacefully placate them using negotiation and/or your emergency salami. Nothing works; physical conflict appears inevitable. But with your toupee, you can harness the element of surprise and murder them legally under the guise of self-defense, thanks to Florida's "Stand Your Ground" law.

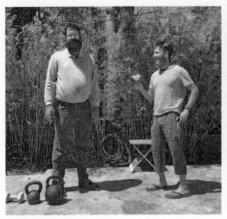

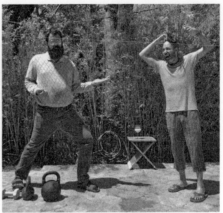

STEP ONE:
Attempt diplomacy. Try to compliment your harasser on their jeans, sandals, or cool shirt.

STEP TWO:
If diplomacy fails, tell long story about Coachella while discreetly using tiny spray bottle of alcohol to loosen toupee glue. Be careful to avoid spraying in your eyes, as this may cause blindness. Also, make sure there is adequate ventilation to avoid inhaling fumes, as this may cause death.

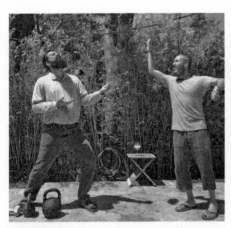

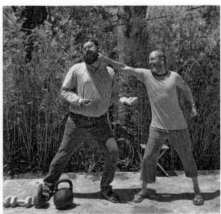

STEP THREE:
Once toupee is loose, tear if off your head and throw it in the air. Attacker's eyes will follow the toupee.

STEP FOUR:
Use this "window of distraction" to step forward and punch them in the face.

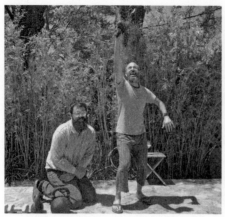

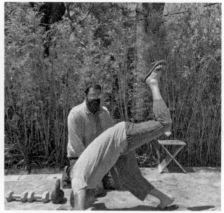

STEP FIVE:
As they fall to the ground, catch your toupee.

STEP SIX:
Somersault behind them, or if there isn't a
gym mat on the floor, simply walk.

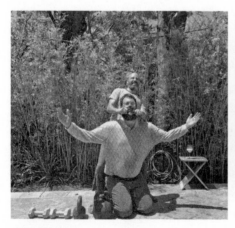

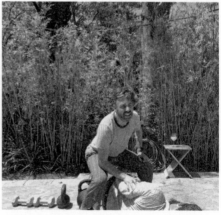

STEP SEVEN:
Grab your toupee by the ends. Pull it over their
mouth and nose. Choke 'em out!

STEP EIGHT:
Put toupee back on and abandon corpse. Any
witness will say the murder was committed
by a bald man and you have hair (remount
backward for extra witness confusion)!

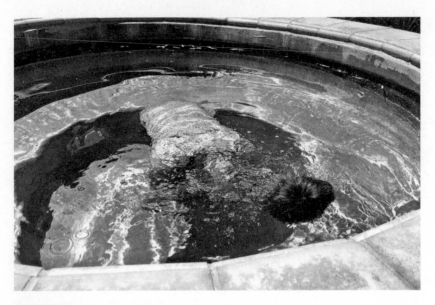

STEP NINE:
Escape into nearby hot tub. How could they possibly catch you?

Now that I had hair again, it was time to reenter society.

The first thing I did was post my new photo and résumé on LinkedIn. No sooner had I clicked UPLOAD than I had my first surprise—my INBOX began filling up with opportunities. I always thought LinkedIn was just a Ponzi scheme for people to dick around and pretend to work—and for bald guys, it is. But just ten minutes before, a job as a CEO, CFO, CTO, submarine commander, or thoracic surgeon seemed like an impossibility. Walking out on my wife and two children would never have occurred to me. But now, I was questioning everything I'd ever held as sacred: "Why not leave my family?" "Who says shoplifting is wrong?" "Why can't you have eggs for dinner?" Baldness was no longer tethering me to complacent behavior. A whole new world opened before me, and I intended to take advantage.

In addition to the smiles I was now routinely getting around town, I also couldn't believe how much small talk I had to make now that I had a piece. No one wants to talk when you're bald. There were whole months I communicated solely with pointing and deep sighs. But now, suddenly, I was forced to sit and smile while everyone babbled at me about nothing. I felt like Ryan Seacrest.

As positively as strangers reacted—these were people who had no idea I'm actually bald, of course—people who knew me reacted violently and negatively to my "hair." "I hate that!" "Take that rug off your head!" "Get off our ski slope, you bald Jew!!"

Where could this hostility be coming from? Why would they care that I had done something good for myself? It took a lot of pondering, but I finally stumbled on what I think the answer is.

I think it's this: We balds, and our baldness, are something people are able to point to as examples of "at least I'm not that!" We are how they justify whatever negative is going on in their lives—they can always say "At least I'm not *bald like him*." If their reliably bald friend suddenly gets hair, then maybe these people have to look more closely at their own shortcomings. Maybe they *are* failures. And their egos can't handle it, so they want us to go back to being ABAP (As Bald as Possible) ASAP.

There's an ugly slur bandied about by those who've lived life with no follicular opposition. They secretly call us people with toupees "nouveau hair." They say we're "gauche" and "boorish." "Old Hair" feels that they are entitled to it all—symphony tickets, the best seats at restaurants, going first at tetherball—as an endless army of deferential bald people serves them caviar and canapés with a "yes, ma'am, yes, sir," then whisks their wet, balled-up napkins away. But then we with "nouveau hair" show up, and the Old Hairsters can't stand the way we turn things on their literal heads, pulling up in our Porsches, our glued-on authentic human hair from Thailand ruffling in the breeze. "Old Hair doesn't need to show hair, we hide it!" they whisper, clutching their pearls and hats with fake fruit on top.

Old Hair believes their hair is some divine seal of approval, proof of genetic superiority and strength of character. They believe the world bending to them isn't coincidence, it's merit. They think, in summary, their good fortune isn't *luck*, it's *skill*.

But if hair isn't a sign of providence—if it can be (God forbid) *purchased*—if millions of years of breeding and heritage, producing fulsome locks, can be replaced in a minute by imported Asian follicles, glue, and tape, then their whole world crumbles, and they'll be buried by rubble at the center of it all. And rightfully, it scares the shit out of them.

Just as gay rights advocates screamed, "We're here! We're queer! Get used to it!" we hairpiece-wearers should shout from the rooftops, "I have a toupee! It's on display! I may or may not be gay! Get used to it!"

Well, fuck my family and friends and Old Hair—the rest of the world was loving my rug.

One of the guys I'd connected with on LinkedIn, Jake, invited me for an interview. As he told me over three cans of an energy drink called Bro Juice, his company had recently been torn apart by a sex scandal and all the men except him had been fired. They needed to restaff quickly, but no women would work there after what happened, so for just this once they were recruiting people like me, white men with an Ivy League degree. I couldn't believe my luck!

It was such a rad meeting. There we were, two guys with hair and thick gold chains bonding over golf courses, grilling, and a shared passion for corporate synergy. Then Jake threw kind of a curveball and asked, "What's your greatest weakness?" I knew I was at a crossroads. My greatest weakness is, of course, my toupee. But I couldn't be New Hair in an Old Hair world. I smiled, ran my fingers through my mane, and said, "Well, if anything I guess I spend too much time styling my hair." Jake laughed. "I would too if I were you. You're hot, brother!" He extended his hand and the job was mine. On the way out, he grabbed my ass. I was gonna like this place!

So there I was, an associate VP at a company I can't name, for legal reasons. Our mission was to provide "integrated solutions for a virtual world." I didn't really know what that meant, and no one else seemed to either. It's amazing how far you can get just by saying "But will it scale?" and "We need to loop in Dennis before we make a move."

For the bald man, time doesn't fly, it crawls. All of life seems too long. Wearing a hairpiece, days started to zing by like they did when I was young. I was busy with meetings, presentations, looping in Dennis, and a secret heterosexual underwear wrestling club with Jake and a few of the other guys, and I damn near felt immortal. Whether it was the hair or toxic levels of Bro Juice or some combination thereof, who knows?

I was so absorbed, for the first time since 2001, I didn't spend even a second worrying about my hair. Everything was how I imagined my best life could be—a corporate job, sweet khakis, four friends named Scott. Talking to colleagues and clients, we were now on equal hair footing. In fact, I started to feel like when I talked to bald people, *I* was doing *them* a favor. I was starting to have hair privilege. And I *loved* it.

But I was leading a double life—hair during the day, then every night at home, the curtains safely shut, I'd remove the toupee and go through the agony of balding all over again. Like Cinderella's chariot, my head would turn back into a pumpkin. All the rage, anxiety, and agony I thought I was done suffering would reappear, only even more intensely every time I removed it.

There were now two me's: Bald Me and Hair Me. Bald Me was a devoted father. Hair Me saw raising kids as women's work. Bald Me was courteous, deferential, and considerate almost to the point of supplication. Hair Me could care less and used the word "biznich" a lot.

I liked Hair Me precisely because Hair Me was so unlikable. All the annoying neediness I developed as a bald man vanished. But there was a downside too—I started noticing all the other things wrong with me I never noticed when I was bald: My teeth were yellow. My nose was lopsided. I was starting to get man-boobies.

Then, one morning as I was gelling my toupee, I looked down at my hand in horror—hairs! The toupee had begun to shed! Now my real head and my fake head were both going bald.

It was the worst of all worlds—the problems of the haired man and the bald man all at once. The lie of the hairpiece had emboldened me to tell bigger and bigger lies about myself, creating a sick circle of deception. I couldn't remember who I'd told what about whom. I'd promised several people a lift to Boca on a jet I didn't own, and others a private audience with rebel billionaire Richard Branson. I couldn't even remember which lies I was telling myself. I continued to wear it, but my life, like my toupee, was starting to come apart.

My toupee was still fooling everyone except a coworker we called "Bald Scott" (because he was bald). I couldn't quite be sure if he was on to me or not. He'd stare a little long after all our interactions and he seemed to work the word "seam" into every conversation. Had he spotted the telltale overlap around the sides of my head? And if so, would he expose me? Was he a potential ally to confide in, or a threat to be neutralized?

I ran some game theory on the scenario. If I confided in Bald Scott, he could either keep the secret or destroy me. But even if he kept the secret, he could then use it to blackmail me. And even if he didn't blackmail me right away, I'd have to worry about it as long as he was alive. However, if I moved against him, it would be just bald him against me and everyone else with hair. And if I got him first and then he tried to expose me as bald, his accusations would just look like vindictive, desperate flailing. There was no upside to preserving Bald Scott and significant downside. I had to take him out.

By passing as haired, I'd learned that there's no limit to the amount of joy people will take at belittling bald guys. Accordingly, I began a subtle campaign to undermine Bald Scott—some light mocking after he left the room and photoshopped pictures of his head on Homer Simpson's body. Then I got everyone together, Dennis, Jake, the other three Scotts. I told them that SalesCon was coming up, and we should nominate Bald Scott to present as a joke, then dump pig's blood on his head. I was way older than everyone else and they'd never seen the movie *Carrie*, so they thought this was an amazing idea.

Bald Scott was flattered when we told him. You could tell it was the best thing ever to happen in his bald life. What a putz.

I did feel a remote pang of guilt, but at that point, my toupee had so clouded my judgment that "right" and "wrong" were whatever I wanted them to be. Having hair was like dealing blackjack instead of playing. From the other side of the table, the person enjoying himself, sipping "free drinks," doubling down, hitting, and staying is just a rube who will eventually lose.

It was the night before SalesCon and everything was in place. I had bought several pints of what I was pretty sure was pig's blood off of Craigslist. Fifteen other branches of the company had flown in and everyone would witness Bald Scott's humiliation.

And then, it got more complicated.

I was at home, in the shower, blissfully detailing my nutsack with a sable brush and Neatsfoot oil when there was a knock on the bathroom door.

Bald Scott entered. My wife had let him in. Apparently, the night before, she'd grabbed my phone and found all the pictures from Secret Heterosexual Underwear Wrestling Club and recognized Scott immediately. I had stupidly hidden them in a folder called "Secret Heterosexual Underwear Wrestling Club." She said, "If this is what you want, you can have it!" and slammed the door, waking the baby.

I was standing there, and Bald Scott could see everything: my bald head, and my penis. I froze and we stared at each other for what seemed like twenty minutes, because it was twenty minutes.

Finally, he said, "I know." Since I didn't know if he meant he knew about the plans to dump pig's blood on his head and have it go viral and pivot the company to a prank show or he knew about me being bald, I decided to play it cool.

"You know *what*?" I asked, and took a giant gulp of my shower beer.

"I know you're bald."

"What gave it away?"

"The seam. You have to know it's the first thing every bald guy notices."

"Of course I do," I replied. "Well, what do you want from me?" I asked, figuring maybe two hundred grand would shut this thing down.

Bald Scott then surprised me. "Nothing," he said. "I could sense it getting weird with us the last few weeks. Unfortunately, I know all too well how hard it is losing your hair, and I just want to say, man-to-man, your secret's safe with me."

I'd like to say my heart warmed to him at this moment, but Hair Me was still plotting. Even if Bald Scott was bullshitting me, I quickly calculated it was better to at least have the chance that he was on my side than make an enemy for sure.

He picked up my toupee off the sink and held it up to the light, examining it. "Doesn't it suck being bald?" he said. I agreed it did. Bald Scott and I finished showering together in uneasy silence.

SalesCon was amazing, as you can imagine. All the regional offices were there, there was a huge banner, and there was so much shrimp. Between the glad-handing and crustaceans, I had no time to be un-nerved by Bald Scott's visit the night before. And as the time for his presentation approached, I felt no remorse. I actually felt a sense of peace and belonging, the way people with hair undoubtedly do all the time.

It felt good to be part of a team. It felt good to be part of a company, even if I still had no idea what we did. My toupee had brought me to this moment, and if all I had to do was sacrifice one bald man at the altar for the gods to anoint me to corporate greatness, was that so bad?

I had achieved so much in just a month of having hair. It had convinced me that if I wasn't bald, I'd be Tom Cruise, John Legend, or the president. I know this because I'm definitely the best actor in the world, I'm amazing at karaoke, and I'm the smartest person I've ever met. I've literally never met a single person who's better at anything than I am, and the only possible explanation for my relative lack of success is baldness.

This may come as a shock to you, but the world is not a level playing field. The fix is in for people with hair. In an ideal world, we'd take physical appearance out of the equation, so people would have to sink or swim on talent or character alone. But that's not the world we live in. And at some point in his life, every man has to pick a side: Underdog or majority? Good or evil? Hair or bald?

Seeing Bald Scott crying and covered in pig's blood, my answer became clear.

As the cackling grew louder and the jeering more cruel, I was like the Spaniard at the bullfight who suddenly grasps that the real animal isn't the gored bull, it's the braying crowd. Those guffawing dickheads were the same people who, for years prior, wouldn't employ me, date me, or even talk to me because I was bald. They wouldn't stop with Bald Scott. Next week it would be a different target—someone else who was too bald or too ethnic or too effeminate or just too much of an individual to be another joiner pointing and laughing at a victim of cruelty.

There is a huge difference psychologically between actually having hair and having a piece of mesh covered with authentic human hair in a drawer you keep with a bunch of spare keys and all of your sex toys from past relationships. I may have been able to fool other people with my toupee, but I couldn't fool the most important person of all: myself.

Most people have one great lost love. For bald men, the "one who got away" is their hair. And once she took me back, we had both changed too much for it to work.

I could no more go back to hair any more than I could move back into my parents' house and live in my old room. I've learned too much, come too far, and that world is too small. Also, my dad is dead and the people who bought the old house bulldozed it and put up a McMansion that's way out of my price range.

In becoming bald, I had become vulnerable, weak, and ashamed, but in becoming vulnerable, weak, and ashamed, something of value had happened—I had begun to understand that others are also vulnerable, weak, and ashamed, and rather than view them with scorn, I developed something I'd never had before: compassion. And this compassion was, hair or not, the best thing about me.

I never liked Bald Scott, and I knew I couldn't make it better, but there was one way I could make it stop. I strode to the podium, grabbed the microphone, and yelled, "Hey! You think baldness is funny?! Well, then maybe this is funny!" Then I grabbed my toupee and ripped it off.

The crowd gasped as they saw their associate VP, colleague, and friend with the great hair was actually—horror of horrors—bald. I realized, in the adrenaline rush, I had forgotten it was glued on and had torn all the skin off my head as well. I was now balder than I'd ever been, down to the bloody skull. The screaming and chortling was now at my expense, and I was blinded by the light of a thousand cellphones filming me. In that moment, I found a new identity in their laughter, not in who I was, but in who I wasn't. I wasn't them and I never would be.

As baldness had alienated me from my original self, the toupee had alienated me from my bald self and now, in front of everyone yet completely alone, I freefell down into nothing. I may not have known who I was any longer, but I finally knew what I had to do.

22

Loving Someone Bald

By this point, you've hopefully implemented my techniques, seen massive gains in happiness, and amassed new levels of wealth. I know so many of you learned to read just for this book and you've earned a break.

So take this chapter off. Crack a malt liquor for yourself and hand the book to your spouse, girlfriend, parents, stepparents, siblings, friends, boss, coworkers, and clergy, so they can learn more about how to better love, nurture, and cherish you. Let them know how important it is to you that they read this chapter. In five minutes, text them, "Have you read it yet?" If they say no, keep texting them every five minutes until they say they have. Then text, "Wasn't it fascinating what he said about rabbits?" If they agree it was, then you know they are a fucking liar and you need to cut them out of your life immediately.

Dear Bald Lover or Associate,

Baldness doesn't just destroy the man who is bald—it also creates a ripple effect that ruins marriages, obliterates relationships, and tears families apart. Everyone either knows someone bald or is bald themselves. A staggering statistic: Baldness affects more people than cancer and trapeze accidents combined.

Obviously, not being bald, your thoughts are infected by "hair privilege" and you need to check this immediately. Simply know that all your opinions about everything are stupid and invalid and bald people have every right to yell at you and hate you. I hate you. Don't defend yourself, that's hair privilege. I don't want to hear any lip from you or I will turn this book around and we will go home.

How do you eradicate hair privilege? Two ways: Go bald, or die. Anything else is just words.

This book has been one-sided so far. It has focused on ways in which the bald man gets you, the haired person, to be his friend, lover, mate, coworker, clergyman, or relative. Time to turn the tables. Why are you pursuing a bald man? Are you nefarious, desperate, or simply bald-curious? I'm not sure what your angle is here, you sick fuck, but let's go.

How do we understand the bald man? What makes him tick? Or tock? Or tic? Or talk?

Bald men serve many functions in our society: fathers, brothers, sons, sisters, lovers, knights, wizards, clerics, apothecaries, blacksmiths, stable boys, friends, beacons in a storm. Despite your best efforts to avoid them, you will frequently encounter baldies, whether they're taking your change at a tollbooth, selling you a used stereo, or indicting your mother for perjury. Some of you may have won a bald man in a high-stakes game of pai gow poker. We're everywhere and we're not going away. You may have one in your house right now.

If you notice that a friend, relative, or lover is going bald, email me immediately. Anyone else going bald is the best possible news for all bald men, especially if they're even balder than I am. Don't judge me, you hair-privilege turd.

The most important thing you need to know about dealing with a bald man is it's like holding a frog in your hand, and not just because frogs are also bald. The bald man is constantly terrified. His heart rate never drops below 180. You must be very tender and gentle with the bald man, or he will fear-urinate all over you. Experience has taught us there are threats everywhere, so it's best if we remain completely still until whoever is looking at us goes away. Like the frog, he's seen some of his buddies get squished crossing a four-lane highway, and it's burned into his memory. He has every reason to believe you'll turn on him, cheat on him, or bamboozle him, because let's be honest, you probably will.

The bald man's ever-present fears may lead to bouts of temperamental behavior. We are very prone to behavioral extremes: rage, depression, and mania. Occasionally, a feral bald will undergo a complete psychotic break and enter "rampage mode," where he attempts to steal a fire engine and drive it through a mall. It's unclear what triggers this, but once he's lost his marbles and gone "berserker," it's extremely unlikely he'll ever return to reality. Trapping him, then releasing him in the foothills of Denali, if possible, is the most humane thing to do, but for the safety of the community it's probably better to simply blast him at close range with an antiaircraft gun.

Because they are desperately seeking logical order in a world that seems senseless, bald people are also very vulnerable to conspiracy theories. We believe that it's perfectly possible that the Illuminati control the world because every day *we're* controlled by people with hair. If I can lose my hair, isn't it also possible O. J. Simpson was framed? If Nicolas Cage's hair is fake, why can't the moon landing also be fake? Maybe 9/11 was an inside job, and so is LeBron James's hairline. The bald would love nothing more than to have the dark star Nibiru hit the earth and blow everything to smithereens, because in the postapocalyptic rubble we could tell everyone "See? Now you know how we feel."

Given the psychological strain bald men are already under, it's particularly important not to overburden them. Merely getting out of bed, putting on clothes, and facing the outside world can be overwhelming to the hairless. That's why we should never be expected to do chores or yard work, cook, clean, plaster a wall, share with a child, or pay taxes. Those duties should fall to anyone who has hair, and honestly, it's a small price to pay for enduring our not in life.

Living with a bald man may require a complete recalibration of your norms. Bald men are largely nocturnal because we can sunburn in seconds on warm days, or near a 40-watt bulb indoors. Given our inability to partake of daylight, we require a large, warm rock to preserve our core temperature. Our heads grow larger as part of an evolutionary process to prevent our main predator, pythons, from eating us whole. Snake owners will have to choose between having a bald man or a python. We cannot coexist.

Bald men require companionship, but as this book has shown, we find it extremely hard to obtain. It can be helpful to set up "playdates" for your bald man with other bald men. Two strange bald men can find plenty in common, even if they don't speak the same language! One of my best friends is a Nigerian bald who doesn't speak any English and doesn't need to. We both get it—life sucks and we should punch each other until we black out.

You may have seen packs of bald men roaming your town after dusk, communicating via a strange blend of clicks, clacks, high-pitched squeals, and Tagalog. This is a form of pidgin that's been passed down from the ancient balds. Mostly, we're just exchanging advice on where to find friendly sanctuary as we migrate south for winter, but sometimes the information could be vital to preserving our safety. For example, "Ayn yakuk kulai Louis click clack WA-HOO! frepro Empire State Building!" means "A giant hawk just flew off with Louis in its beak and now it's headed for the Empire State Building, WAHOO!"

Like animals, bald men have a sixth sense for when disaster is about to strike. Natural selection has taught us we will be the first people left behind in an earthquake, wildfire, plague of locusts, or other act of God. The bald will "soul-sense" approaching doom for up to twenty minutes before there is even a rumble. If you ever see a wild pack of bald men running in any direction while screaming in bald pidgin/Tagalog, join them! You are likely about to be hit with an earthquake or tsunami. Either that, or someone's giving away free Twix.

Romancing the Bald

People end up with bald men in one of two ways:

1. **Involuntary**—You were involved with someone who wasn't bald, who then went bald and now you're stuck.

2. **Voluntary**—Your life got so bad, you were desperate and made a regrettable choice.

Whether you're a #1 or a #2, you may find yourself wanting to end the relationship. The good thing about breaking up with a bald man is he definitely knows it's coming. We're always prepared for someone to leave us. It's happened so many times, we expect it and make it super easy for you. You won't even need to say the words "We need to talk." As soon as "We" is uttered, we'll fill in the blanks, pack our underwear, sunscreen, dried fruit, emergency salami, and go. It makes dating a bald man very low risk, but it also makes it hard if you intend to stay with him. You have to avoid the word "we" the rest of your life because every time you say it, he's programmed to throw everything into a one-gallon Ziploc and leave.

If you elect to stay in the relationship, there are several benefits to dating an armadillo head.

Unlike regular men, bald men love holding your purse. We know you'll never leave without your purse, so holding it is insurance against being abandoned. I treasure every moment clutching my wife's handbag, because it's at least a few more minutes she'll definitely stay with me. It may be worth marrying us simply as a portable pocketbook caddy. Added bonus: Use your bald man as a handy coatrack! Just toss your jacket on his head. This frees up your arms to make grand sweeping gestures while you describe to someone why another one of your friends is a complete bitch.

Also, we will murder for you. Each bald man is like your own tiny Manchurian candidate. He can be easily programmed to do anything, thanks to his toxic mix of low self-esteem and insatiable craving for approval. In between purse-carrying and assassination, there's obviously a lot of middle ground, which I don't plan to cover here.

While you may regard the bald as so much human flotsam, you can exploit his worthlessness to your advantage. Like back rubs? Demand endless amounts. Want jewels? Make him steal them—not hard, because remember, he's effectively invisible. The only thing a bald man may be hesitant to do is 69. This is because we're self-conscious about having less hair than your vagina. If you're waxed or shaved, we feel less shame, so please never sport anything longer than a half-Brazilian.

Of course, it will be incredibly humiliating for people to find out you're with a bald man. Tongues will flap and rumors will swirl and you may feel you were better off alone. The good news is, no one has to know. He'll totally get why you don't want to tell anyone you're dating him and be fine with it. Just leave him at home for events (better yet, have him give you a ride!), then tell everyone he's really busy so couldn't make it again. Or don't! They won't remember who he is, so they won't care.

You never have to worry about a bald guy cheating on you. He can't—who else is going to jump in the sack with him? Your mere presence in his life is a miracle. You may think dogs and cats are loyal, but some run away the first chance they get. (We've all seen posters on the street lamenting a "Lost Dog"—believe me, there's no such thing as a "lost" dog. They know exactly where they're going—they just don't like you.)

Bald guys are not dogs. You could release a bald man into the Sahara, come back eight years later, and he'd be standing in the exact same spot, holding your purse and praying for your return. I'm sure you've seen the YouTube video of "Christian and the Lion" in which a lion joyfully jumps all over Christian after a year apart? That's nothing compared to what I do to my wife every night when she gets home from work. She has a smock she wears whenever I'm around to protect her "good clothes."

Like dogs, when you leave the house, the bald man has no idea when or if you'll return. We lack any concept of time and any faith that you're not out hooking up with guys or women with hair while you're away. And sadly, if you did, on every level we'd understand, because in your shoes we'd do exactly the same thing. As you approach the door to exit, we will likely get agitated, bark in pidgin, and start sprinting in tiny circles.

This emotional intensity can be hard to take every day, so like my wife, you may want to keep an oar handy and bash us in the head to get a brief respite from the bald man's overzealous affections. There are also specialized trainers who will work with a bald man and teach him to sit still when a door opens—they charge upwards of $500 an hour, but it's worth every penny. In my case, it only took thirty sessions to learn to heel. It's probably cheaper and easier to just throw a Twix in the corner and run out while he chases it.

Parenting the Bald

Shame on you! Shame, shame, shame!

You should have known better! You had the bald gene, but you just had to have sex, didn't you, you selfish jackanapes! This whole thing—your bald son's entire tortured future existence—is your fault! All you had to do was either be a virgin forever or get sterilized, but you just couldn't do it, could you, you bum!

I don't want to hear your self-pitying chorus of "Wah-wah, my friends always talk about their children's hair and I can never join in!" If I was in charge, anyone who knowingly passed on the baldness gene would be tarred and feathered, then drawn and quartered, then repaved.

You want to help your poor baldo son? Stop asking when he's moving out. He's not. You have no right to ask or expect him to leave the house. The world has nothing for him. He should be allowed to live in his room and do whatever he wants on the Internet for as many decades as he wants to be there. If anything, *you* should move out. It's way easier for you to start over and build a new life than him. And for God's sake, go get sterilized!

23

Employing the Bald

Bald people make great employees. Devoid of relationships, and jettisoned by society at large, their jobs are all they have.

When you go into the military, the first thing they do is shave your head. Why? Because battlefields are hell on hairstyles, sure, but also to humiliate you, subjugate you, show you that you're now nothing. The army knows that a bald person is a hundred times more likely to run into enemy bullets, because they have no life to speak of. The bald man is, quite simply, preshaved cannon fodder.

Whatever industry you're in, you likewise may well require the work of thousands of loyal, uncreative drones. Balds are ideal for these positions.

And yet, every day, jobs that should be going to Qualified Bald Men (QBMs) in many cases go to women or minorities. And if you point this out to a group of women or minorities, they get angry and call you "racist" or "sexist" instead of instantly giving you their job. It's like people have never heard of "baldlisting"! And baldlisting doesn't just happen in

Hollywood—it also happens in Studio City, Van Nuys, and even as far out as Calabasas.

How did I uncover the bald list? I applied for a consulting job, then ten minutes later applied for the same job wearing a Jennifer Aniston wig. Unfortunately, I got the job both times and had to Mrs. Doubtfire it for the next eight years. At my goodbye party, nine guys made a drunk pass at "Jen."

Bald men love the office. Work is the only place good-looking people talk to us, because they have to. That makes us eager to chat about work *all* the time. For us, there's nothing better than work events, softball games, or retreats, because it's a glimpse at what it's like to have friends who aren't total losers. The fact that everyone else is making 80 percent more than us is a small price to pay for companionship.

Unlike most men, balds love working for women. We have the greatest appreciation for female humans because we have the least access. Sexism is a luxury we can't afford. Work may be the only place women talk to us, so we are polite, conscientious, deferential, and unfailingly loyal. Whereas a regular man with hair is often resistant to female management, a bald guy will happily run around doing your bidding, whether you require a piping-hot latte or simply a discreet, reliable office snitch.

It's incredibly unfair, in fact, that balds are included in any negative generalizations about men. Our merits should always be singled out in qualified statements such as: "All men are pigs *except, of course, bald guys.*" "All men think about is sex *except for bald guys, who are preoccupied with their hair loss, funnel cakes, and death.*"

Bald people will never complain no matter how heavy the workload because we know you're looking for the merest pretext to fire us. We'll never report misconduct to HR because, honestly, whose side is HR going to take? A bald guy's? Or someone with hair's? Facts get twisted, reports get fudged, and next thing you know, *we're* packing a box because someone blew their nose on our Raisinets as a joke. I am 0 for 51 in Human Resources actions dating back to 2002. I also recently brought an official complaint about this obvious bias and lost—0 for 52.

For certain occupations, the bald are even preferable to the haired.

We can sell tons of used cars because we have a lifetime of experience pimping our own used heads.

We make the best chefs because there will never be a hair in the food.

We're great on chain gangs because we love togetherness and song.

Bald people also make better doctors. Because they rarely see them, they get extra excited to examine your penis, vagina, and breasts. They will be extremely thorough and miss no lumps, rare in these topsy-turvy times. You can call them anytime day or night, even on holidays, and they will make an emergency house call. They weren't doing anything. And their hair won't fall into your incision, killing you by infection later.

The bald have endless time to hear you complain and worry about your health—in fact, it's the only thing that makes them feel better about themselves. And if, God forbid, you're going to receive bad news—heart disease, lupus, colon stuff—you will be able to think "Well, at least I'm not bald."

Bald people have nowhere to be nights and weekends and always welcome extra work, so they can justify to themselves why they have nowhere to be on nights and weekends. You can expose them to toxic chemicals and they'll look the same after, which has the handy added bonus of preventing them from winning damages in class-action lawsuits.

Bald men can even be in charge. The Steves Jobs and Ballmer, Jeff Bezos, David Geffen; the list of bald titans of industry goes on and on. Put us in a crowded nightclub, we're no one—put us in a boardroom and we're gold. We'll fire anyone—they were never going to like us anyway. We'll take huge risks—we're already half dead. Long conference calls are our lifeblood—it's the only time someone will talk to us on the phone, though we're useless if they want to Skype.

Bald men are not just great businessmen—they are also the most *dangerous* people you can do business with. What's your leverage? What can you take away from us that we haven't already lost? What pain can you make us feel that won't be a joke compared to our daily suffering? Our word also means nothing because we've fallen for the greatest deception—we believed our hair when it said it would stay on top of our heads.

Capitalism is based on the tacit understanding that both parties are negotiating with the fundamental goal of mutual benefit. But the bald man is like the Joker in Batman—his only friend is chaos. The only end we seek is the joy of watching others panic.

I'm not saying bald men are inherently evil, like redheads—redheads are unreachable and irredeemable. The bald man is significantly more emotionally complex than those the French call *les têtes enflammées*. Nothing will ever make us feel better—not drugs, not riches, not even love—so from our perspective there is no transaction that could possibly be to our benefit. People with hair always get the better end of the deal because at both the beginning and end of our dealings, *they have hair*. This is why all of the shrewdest businessmen, attorneys, and bankers are bald. It's also why no matter what your venture is, your negotiating committee should consist mostly of bald men and perhaps one haired "ambassador," just for show.

Bald-on-bald negotiations can be particularly brutal, as neither party has any inclination, motivation, or ability to give an inch. Put two bald men in a boardroom, and when you open the door eight hours later, all you'll see are shredded suits, two skeletons picked completely clean, and a chessboard locked in double checkmate.

If you're an employer and still unconvinced, you should hire bald to take advantage of a simple fact: Wherever we bald guys are, people always assume we work there, so you might as well have us work there.

At concerts, people assume I'm a record executive. At open houses, they assume I'm the real estate agent. At pharmacies, people ask me to point them toward the douche aisle. At hospitals, people think I'm a doctor. On planes, they think I'm a pilot. In court, I'm the judge. At museums, I'm the dork who runs the planetarium. At funeral homes, they assume I'm the director, which is so awesome because then I get to look in the casket as many times as I want.

Being mistaken for an employee can be annoying for sure, but the real fun starts when you embrace it and stop denying you work there.

This has broadened my perspective considerably. I have performed two total vertex craniectomies and tried a man for murder (not guilty on fifteen counts!). I once docked a Carnival Cruise in Puerto Vallarta. I even starred in two episodes of *Frasier* (Season 9, "Dial N for Niles," and "The Wizard of Roz").

There are tens of millions of ready and eager balds who will do jobs no one else wants to do for less money. They're too scared to ever complain or ask for time off or a raise. They are ready to be exploited and driven past their mental and physical breaking points, solely to help your business succeed. And that's what capitalism is all about! Hire bald!

24

Skinspirations

As a bald man, it's important to surround yourself with bald-positive role models. These fellow cantaloupe heads can provide inspiration to keep battling no matter how bald things seem. They are living (and in some cases dead) proof that you can triumph over hairlessness. Even though none of them would agree to talk to me, these remarkable onion skulls are my personal bald idols. I call them "skinspirations." They are truly heroes, and yes, I *do* use that word lightly.

Pitbull

You never notice that Pitbull is bald because he's always surrounded by a cloud of dry ice. He's basically a mediocre rapping fog monster. It's a true innovation in hiding hair loss: Always be obscured in a cloud of thick condensation, and/or a thick cloud of anger caused by naming yourself after a dog that's best known for attacking children.

Fog is the great equalizer because no one can see you. You could be tall, short, fat, thin, but no one has any idea. That's why bald people should live in London if possible. Prince William and Prince Charles have managed to stay in power precisely because it's foggy in London each August through the following July. We in the U.S., with our access to TMZ and the *National Enquirer*, know they're bald, but the Brits have no idea. If the clouds ever broke, the U.K. would morph instantly from constitutional monarchy to a banana republic.

The Rock

I love The Rock. He's always positive. He's genuinely funny. And he's a really good actor, except in most of his movies.

Fifteen years ago, I went to the gym on a Friday night at 10 P.M., because I was a bald loser with nothing to do. Who was the only other person at Gold's that night, squatting what looked to be 5,000 pounds? The Rock. I said, "Hi, The," and he said, "Please don't talk to me while I'm lifting."

Few know that The Rock isn't bald genetically. He shaves his head because, as he tweeted on April 3, 2017, "I'm not bald because I went bald. I'm bald because my hair is a cross between an afro and hair from a Lama's [*sic*] ball sac [*sic*]." While I question the wisdom of the decision (and I find it distressing he doesn't know how to spell "sack," not to mention "llama"), I respect the hell out of it. The Rock has chosen to be one of us, simply because, like lifting weights, it's difficult and makes you stronger.

I admire him so much, I'm trying to turn myself into a tiny version of The Rock called "The Pebble."

Winston Churchill and Dwight Eisenhower

Winston Churchill inspired Great Britain to persevere through the darkest days of German bombing in World War II, saying things like "We shall defend our island, whatever the cost may be, we shall fight on the beaches, we shall fight on the landing grounds, we shall fight in the fields and in the streets, we shall fight in the hills; we shall never surrender." Of course, Churchill was willing to be bombed into oblivion—he was bald and had nothing to lose.

While grand appeaser Neville Chamberlain was willing to give Europe to Hitler—because that's the type of wink-and-a-handshake deal people with hair have been making since the beginning of time—Churchill wouldn't cede an inch. Why would he? Hitler could never possibly offer the only thing Churchill would want: his hair back.

Similar bald obstinacy led to victory on D-Day. Who but a bald man like Dwight Eisenhower would have the audacity to conceive the idea to storm a beach and rappel up a cliff to fight a fortified enemy? This takes a particular disregard for human life that can only be cultivated by not having hair. And yet no-hair Eisenhower never quite gets the credit he deserves because no-legs Roosevelt sucks up all the kudos. Churchill and Eisenhower are the true heroes. Instead of calling it World War II, we should call it World War B, and the B should stand for "Bald."

Jimmy Buffett

No one thinks of Jimmy Buffett as bald—they think of him as drunk, stoned, and passed out in a hammock. This is a terrific example of strategic misdirection. During an avalanche, no one notices a zit on your nose. Similarly, when you're playing the steel drums and cater-wauling about cheeseburgers, an entire blotto audience won't notice you're bald.

Smartly, Jimmy Buffett branded his fans as "Parrotheads," convincing them they're a fraternity of fun-loving, sea-sailing pirate-people, too rebellious to live by society's rules. In reality, they're just doofuses in Crocs who are dating their stepsister, but people buy into the illusion all the same. Jimmy's not a sun-stroked, inebriated bald boob—he's the life of the party! You're not on Lipitor and have to carry your own oxygen; you're an eccentric, untamable buccaneer! The people who work at the resort don't want to kill you! They love serving you frozen margaritas while they live next to an open sewer!

Liking cheeseburgers and margaritas is in no way interesting or special. Neither is liking vacations and boats. Or the ocean and sex. But write a song like "Why Don't We Get Drunk and Screw?" and suddenly you've convinced people you invented soused humping, when everyone knows that was Susan B. Anthony.

A similar transformation for you could be just a couple wardrobe tweaks and one mediocre song away. Put on a captain's hat and Hawaiian shirt, write a tune about "Grillin' and Fuckin'," and you're no longer a bald, dad-bod doofus—you're a star!

The Dalai Lama, aka "His Baldiness"

A good tactic to shift focus off the loss of your hair is to cultivate the air of an above-it-all swami. It conveys to the world "Am I bald? Huh, wow. I'm so spiritual I didn't even notice. We are all one, by the way."

His Hairlessness sucks at parallel parking and the Chinese government wants to kill him, but he doesn't have to hold down a day job, he's friends with mucho celebs, and even his simplest utterances are taken as profound, life-changing maxims. For example, the Dalai Lama once said, "Remember, that sometimes not getting what you want is a wonderful stroke of luck." Sure, okay, but sometimes it sucks. I'm starving. I want food. There is none. Oh, how lucky!

Still, he gets to hang out with Demi Moore without even marrying her, and he wears his pajamas everywhere. I respect the hustle.

Dennis Franz

The most Chicago thing ever, Dennis Franz was conceived when the Sears Tower mated with the ivy-covered outfield wall at Wrigley Field, which then birthed a middle-aged bald baby who looks like a talking ulcer. Dennis Franz looks how we all feel, like a cop who's way behind on alimony payments and pursuing a serial killer he'll never catch. He's never been old or young, he's always just been annoyed.

No one would look at that face and body and think, "He should be a huge TV star," and yet that sonofabitch pulled it off, making America fall in love with the racist, alcoholic Andy Sipowicz. I think about Dennis Franz a lot and hope he's happy, but no way he is. I mean, look at him.

Scott Kelly

Scott Kelly is a bald astronaut who holds the record for longest NASA mission after spending 340 days straight on board the International Space Station. Or at least that's what the CIA wants us to think.

From John Glenn to Story Musgrave to Scott Kelly, America has shown a great willingness to launch bald people into space as disposable explorers. Due to balds' willingness to blow up on a launch pad or asphyxiate to death at any moment, we make the ideal payload for any long-distance capsule. Mark my words: When the first human being sets foot on Mars, he will be as bald as Mars itself.

Space and its vast, uncharted frontiers provide the greatest hope to the bald man. From *E.T.* to Yoda to the aliens in *Aliens*, everything indicates that we are not alone in the universe, and that those we share the universe with are bald. Baldness must then be a sign of intelligence that's so far advanced it's beyond man's understanding. Perhaps as we progress on earth, haired people will die off, leaving balds to inherit everything.

I welcome an alien takeover of the world, and you should hope for it as well. In any "War of the Worlds" scenario, I'm picking up a ray gun and mowing down as many humans as possible. You have to assume aliens would come to earth, take a look around, save their fellow bald brethren, and annihilate everyone with hair. God, that would be so sweet! I just hope I live long enough to see everyone from Logan Paul to Phil Michelson obliterated in an inferno.

It's theoretically possible that bald people *are* aliens, the result of E.T.'s visiting earth thousands of years ago and impregnating humans, maybe during their Spring Break. It would explain why bald people feel so separate from the rest of humanity.

Drawings based on the recollections of people who claim to have been abducted always feature bald aliens. These stories of abduction seem to follow roughly the same narrative: Someone was alone, at night, in a rural area of the Deep South. They saw a bright light, lost consciousness, then, next thing they knew, bald extraterrestrials were examining their rectum. Then they were returned to earth, and the aliens promised to call but never did.

Given that, I frequently find myself wandering naked down rural Kentucky roads, hoping a spaceship will appear and whisk me away. They can look in my butt all they want. And take anything you find in there, I'm not using it.

As I wander these dirt roads, lit only by starlight, it's easy to imagine another bald man on another planet, naked and wandering another dirt road, staring at the stars and seeking communion. In these moments, space and time seem less like mathematical concepts and more like a comfortable jacket we're both wearing to stave off the cold until the day we can warm ourselves in one another's embrace. As long as even the idea of a bald man across the cosmos exists, I am never alone.

So far, I have been abducted and had my anus explored several times, not by aliens but by men in pickup trucks wielding shotguns who repeatedly insist they're married to women. I generally see a bright light and lose consciousness, then wake up to find myself covered in bruises. These beautiful nude walks, walks that end with a bourbon waterboarding and car battery torture, are a small price to pay for my pursuit of . . . a final frontier.

Howie Mandel

Probably the best-known practitioner of the old "don't-look-up-there-where-there-is-nothing-just-notice-my-soul-patch-and-diamond earrings" strategy. He has less a face than a jewelry store with a goatee entrance. Howie also claims to be germaphobic, which cleverly makes it seem like not touching anyone is his choice, not theirs.

Andre Agassi

We all know tennis is very stupid. You hit a green ball over a net for no reason. Even though it would be way more fun to crank the ball a billion feet, they make you keep it in between the lines. Each point counts as fifteen, until the third point, which counts as ten. That's so dumb.

Still, as mind-numbing as it is (and again, tennis really is for imbeciles), Andre Agassi played the 1990 French Open final in a wig held together by twenty bobby pins, lost, then publicly admitted he was bald. He dated some of the world's most beautiful women and was even so good at doing meth he almost became addicted. Agassi runs his own educational foundation and seems like a genuinely good person. His success cleared the way for no one bald to be good at tennis since.

Paul Simon

Paul Simon writes gorgeous melodies matched by insightful, poetic lyrics. But early in his career, he knew if he stood onstage by himself, people would say, "Look at that short, bald fuck, singin' like a bird. Siddown, baldy!" So what did he do to become famous? He hired a big, redheaded dork with the incredibly distracting name Garfunkel to stand next to him.

Simon's audiences were too busy laughing at this ridiculous "Garfunkel" to even see the tiny egghead next to him. And Garfunkel, a ginger weirdo, was just happy to be allowed out of the Redheads Only reservation in Wyoming where he was raised. Sure, Paul Simon was forced to give up half the credit, but now he's the greatest living songwriter apart from a bunch of better ones, and he's at least able to stand onstage and sing "Bridge Over Troubled Water" without getting pelted with beer cans.

I love seeing concerts by Paul Simon, Kenny Chesney, or Billy Joel, because as long as they show up, I won't be the baldest guy in the stadium.

William Shakespeare

Bald, and the greatest writer in history. Coincidence? Yes.

Romeo and Juliet—what's a better story than two teenagers killing themselves on a bed? Its moral remains as important today as when it was written: We should let fourteen-year-olds get married. Shakespeare also wrote *Julius Caesar, Hamlet, Othello, Macbeth, King Lear,* and is the reason, to this day, that CliffsNotes remain so popular.

Despite living in the 1500s, Shakespeare was married to Anne Hathaway. Look it up, it's true. She's way older than everyone thinks.

Michael Jordan

Before he became known as the world's premier collector of horrible jeans, Michael Jordan was actually famous as the eighteenth-greatest basketball player of all time. Jordan's signature move was losing a $10,000 blackjack hand at half court, then running down and dunking the ball while carrying two giant stacks of casino chips. Michael Jordan won six NBA championships without hair, a feat that will never be repeated.

Jordan overcame an incredible amount of adversity en route to his professional success. As a sophomore he didn't even make the high school varsity team! This led to three months where he was angry about not making the team as a sophomore, or as everyone who writes about sports calls it, "an incredible amount of adversity." After that, his life was pretty much nonstop acclaim, but still, Jordan harnessed those bad three months and used them to alienate teammates for the next twenty years, which I'm told was incredibly inspiring.

Before Jordan, bald people were widely regarded as losers, but thanks to him, bald people can now also be regarded as asshole winners. It's indisputable that Jordan was super bald and had an incredible will to compete. Michael Jordan's success teaches us it doesn't matter what's on top of your head. The most important organ of the body—the heart—is bald.

25

Matthew McConaughey

No good book is complete without a chapter devoted to Matthew McConaughey. He's the triple axel of writing, a compulsory jump where you'll be judged by both your interpretation and your execution. John Updike struggled with "the McConaughey Question" for decades. The same quagmire tormented J. D. Salinger into isolation and drove Sylvia Plath insane. And yet, here I am.

What you are about to read will shock you to your core. It is a conspiracy that goes from Hollywood all the way up to the White House, and it doesn't even involve sexual harassment. It exposes a stunning web of illicit coordination between the FBI, CIA, ATF, NSA, KGB, FTA, DEA, and even CVS.

Occam's razor is a principle that states that the simplest explanation for events is most often correct. However, there is a corollary, Occam's beard, which states that the most ornate, complex, and illogical theory must also be true. Never has Occam's beard applied more than to what I'm about to tell you, information the government does not want you to know. I even had my life threatened by my own wife, although she claims it was unrelated. In any case, you should probably tell someone you are about to read this, so if you show up dead, they'll know it's a murder.

FACT:

In 1999, neighbors called the police with a noise complaint. When the police arrived, they found Matthew McConaughey, nude and playing the bongos. A mug shot was taken with this dilapidated, eroding-beach hairline.

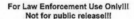

For Law Enforcement Use Only!!!
Not for public release!!!

Austin Police Department   Page: 1

Intel #: 1998-31503

PD Number: 367396

Person: MCCONAUGHEY, MATTHEW DAVID   DOB:/ /   Sex: Race:

Alias:

By: GONZALES   TC330   10/25/1999 11:58   By: GONZALES   TC330   10/25/1999 11:59

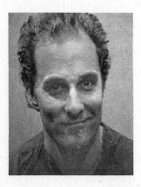

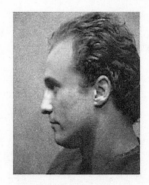

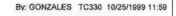

FACT:

In the years 1999 to 2009, Matthew McConaughey was a mediocre actor with a receding hairline who appeared in such bland romantic comedies as *The Wedding Planner, How to Lose a Guy in 10 Days,* and *Ghosts of Girlfriends Past.*

FACT:

In 2010, no Matthew McConaughey movies were released. No one cared.

FACT:

In 2011, Matthew McConaughey returned with *a full head of hair* in *The Lincoln Lawyer,* beginning a string of acclaimed performances where he has gone from a milquetoast, thinning-hair supporting actor to a fully maned Oscar-winning star. These movies include incredible turns in *The Wolf of Wall Street, Magic Mike,* and *Dallas Buyers Club,* and he was also terrific in the first season of *True Detective,* which I saw before my brother changed his HBO GO password.

TO REITERATE:

A balding person of little ability disappeared, grew hair, then returned as one of the greatest actors of our time. How did this happen? Are you ready to go down the rabbit hole?

THEORY:

The original, balding Matthew McConaughey was eliminated by the CIA and replaced by a doppelgänger with hair who can act.

Shocking, *n'est-ce pas?*

Well, how do we know the Matthew McConaughey today isn't just the original Matthew McConaughey in a hairpiece? That's easy: The original one couldn't act, whereas the haired one can. People don't just suddenly become good at acting at age forty. And he's not the only instance of a literal Hollywood bigwig I believe has been replaced because they're balding. I can't print the photos here for risk of assassination, but go to Google and verify the following:

In the 1990s, Ben Affleck was a writer with a bald spot. In the early 2000s, he became a hirsute movie star. Jamie Foxx, hairline-receding comic actor, suddenly sprouts a full head of hair and an Oscar for *Ray*. Jeremy Piven: balding and middling in *PCU*, then miraculously grew hair and learned how to act for *Entourage*.

There was even an incident where it *didn't* work out. Mel Gibson was clearly replaced around 2005, and sadly the doppelgänger they found was a racist, anti-Semitic drunk. They have since attempted to rehabilitate the fake several times, but he's too religious or inebriated for most people's tastes, and he's never recaptured the magic of the original Mel.

Why is the government eliminating bald bad actors, then replacing them with full-hairline ones who don't chew the scenery?

Movies do more than even sports to spread a positive perception of America worldwide. Having bald stars would make us look weak and open the way for another superpower—say Russia—to steal away the world's hearts by displaying celebrities with thick hair.

But it goes even deeper. Movies are a gigantic business. Most of the studios producing blockbusters are run by international conglomerates. Chinese money, in particular, is propping up the film industry. China is also the largest buyer of U.S. debt, which keeps our entire economy running. And the long-term creditworthiness of U.S. treasuries is mostly based on perception.

If a bald Matthew McConaughey or hairless Mel Gibson were to front a motion picture and it bombed, the ensuing economic loss could endanger not only the studio but Sino-U.S. relations as well. Realizing the financially catastrophic consequences if China stopped purchasing our debt, and having war-gamed a conflict with China and found potential casualties in the tens of millions, I believe the CIA formed the following covert plan: Bald movie stars would be kidnapped and placed on board a jet, a crash faked, and the original Matthew McConaughey, Jamie Foxx, Jeremy Piven, Mel Gibson, and God knows who else are being held on a secret tropical island.

How?

Malaysia Airlines Flight MH370 took off on March 8, 2014, under normal conditions. Fourteen minutes into the flight, the transponder went off, ceasing active communications and disappearing from radar. The plane was never seen or heard from again.

My theory—which has never been refuted by official or unofficial government sources—is that the original actors listed above were on this flight. The government couldn't crash the plane—that would draw too much attention, and the plan might be blown by DNA if the plane was ever found. Besides, what if by some small percentage chance Matthew McConaughey survived? They'd kinda *have* to put him in a movie after that.

The plan was to send the actors to the same atoll where they vanished Amelia Earhart, where, cruelly, their genes, stem cells, and remaining hair plugs are harvested and used to regularly rejuvenate their replacements. Tragically, the other passengers on the flight were simply collateral damage in the centuries-long war on baldness. It's the CIA's ultimate revenge on bald people for what Sinatra did in our name to JFK (see Chapter 12).

But what of the three pieces of debris found from the flight—the wing fragment, wing flap, and flaperon? Those were planted by the CIA to throw us off the scent. We should be searching for that jet as far away from those pieces as possible!

Sound crazy? You're crazy if you think that's *not* what happened. The Tuskegee experiment; MK Ultra, the CIA's secret mind-control project; the bombing of Greenwood in Tulsa, Oklahoma; the Gulf of Tonkin incident; Saddam Hussein's "Weapons of Mass Destruction"; sorry, buttercup, but there are dozens of examples of a shadow government using nefarious means to act in what they think is the country's "best interest."

I guarantee there's an island of bald celebrities who at first were sustaining themselves on coconuts, but now, five years later, are eating one another to survive. Jamie Foxx has probably just devoured Mel Gibson's liver, while Ben Affleck waits in the brush with a crudely shaped spear, ready to impale Mickey Rourke while he sleeps. It's a national shame, and I hope someday it's unmasked, maybe in a hundred years, when they discover a mint-condition plane surrounded by skeletons and iPhone 6's.

Airplanes, like baldness, don't just disappear. Both leave behind a mess that scatters for thousands of miles. Ask yourself, Which is more likely: that Jeremy Piven regrew his hair and learned to act? Or that who we think is Jeremy Piven is not Jeremy Piven at all?

26

What Does It All Mean?

Why are you bald?

I don't mean what makes you biologically not have hair. I mean in the largest possible sense—why would there be a universe, be a you, and then the you is bald? What is the fucking point of all this?

Some of history's greatest thinkers have grappled with the existence of God, as have some of history's worst thinkers. There are many different versions of God, but they all basically boil down to the same thing: an invisible person who gives a shit about what happens to you. Usually, the God is theoretically really awesome and conveniently did a bunch of impossible stuff before anyone had a camera, so we'll have to take some book's word for it.

Typically, these gods are kind of egomaniacs and get off on ruining people's weekends by making them go to an expensive building without enough parking to say how awesome the god is in unison with some other people who only showed up because there are free donuts. When you die, maybe you get to meet the god and see your old dogs and play volleyball and stuff, or maybe you burn in an eternal fire. No one knows, so don't steal stuff or mouth off to your parents. That's religion in a nutshell.

Now that you're completely caught up on theology and eschatology, how does this affect you and your hairlessness? Is it worth your time to join a church or temple and mumble at the sky hoping a god is listening and will help? Here are some things to consider:

If there is a God, he let you go bald. Therefore, he either doesn't care enough to give you hair, or is powerless to do so.

Well, not a great start.

God has made you bald to test you.

Well, why is God testing you and not Blake Shelton? How do you pass this test? By being bald and not being miserable? Presumably, if God controls everything, he's the one who also made you miserable. By not being miserable, you'd be undoing his work. So either God should make thee not bald and miserable, or bald and happy about it!

God didn't make you bald.

Well, you're still bald, so even if it isn't God's fault, she (?) blatantly either isn't powerful enough or doesn't care enough to give you hair. And if a God isn't powerful or caring, why worship them? Also, if God didn't make me bald, then who did? Because I need to know whose ass to kick.

You are created in God's image, and God is bald.

I'm not worshiping a bald guy. And why would God also create people with hair who are better-looking than he is? Is it because God's generous and kind of self-effacing, or because he's bald and hates himself? Or does God actually think baldness looks better, in which case he's either stupid or insane? And if God knows baldness is worse than having hair and still made you bald, it's hard not to take that as kind of a personal fuck you.

God doesn't have a mirror, so he has no idea how he looks.

Maybe he's bald or maybe he has hair; *even he doesn't know.* In this line of reasoning, baldness is then entirely a human construct, like gazebos or Mucinex, so our plight in no way reflects on him. When we worship God, then, we are not worshiping an all-knowing being, which may or may not be a problem, depending on how anal you are about that type of thing.

God has made you bald, but God only gives people as much as they can handle.

Wrong! If you could handle being bald, for starters you wouldn't be reading this book. And why would God provide a concierge service of personally tailored maladies set to precisely your level? Why test people at all? Why not just give them everything and make them all happy?

God exists and is all-powerful but simply has a strong dislike for you so he made you bald.

This one is pretty hard to refute. But prayer hasn't made my hair come back, and if there's nothing I can do to win God back to my side and give me hair, then why even try?

God made you bald, but God also spoke through me to give you this book, which will help you get through being bald.

Hmm. I give this a hard "maybe." I won't be mad at God if this book makes a lot of money. But, if this is true, would it have killed him to help out a little more? He wrote the whole Bible, but for this book he couldn't even kick in a chapter?

Baldness itself is superior in some unrevealed way, which will become apparent at the very moment of death.

That would be so cool, it almost makes me want to die! I'm holding out hope, for sure, but statistically it's just as likely that there is an afterlife and you could be bald in it for eternity. And isn't any heaven that contains baldness not really heaven at all? By definition, heaven by its nature has to be free of baldness, or I'm gonna destroy it on Yelp.

Therefore, to be heaven—i.e., eternal perfection—one of its characteristics must be that you get hair the moment you die. If so, and that's for eternity, I'm not that mad about being bald these next one to fifty years. I don't mind believing in that. Does this make me Presbyterian?

You are already bald and in hell, and one of the properties of hell is that it seems like it's not hell and you have hope and control over your fate. However, you are actually just locked into an eternal cycle of disappointment and anguish for deeds committed in a past life that you can't even remember.

Okay, but if this is hell, then why is there so much delicious pizza?

There is no God and the universe is simply governed by the principles of quantum mechanics, or some other course you got a C-minus in.

According to Heisenberg's uncertainty principle, matter exists in an indefinite state called "duality," which is neither wave nor particle until someone observes it. This is the basis of the famous thought experiment "Schrödinger's cat," where a cat in a box is neither alive nor dead until someone opens the box (either way, it sounds like someone should call the ASPCA).

Likewise, I would posit, in a godless universe, you are neither bald nor have hair until someone looks at you. This would be comforting except that people look at you to determine whether or not they want to have sex with you. Then they see you're bald and decide not to.

Should we all be atheists, then? Well, not so fast, you coastal elite. If there is no God, then who came up with quantum mechanics? They just appeared out of nowhere? If something could come from nothing, then you'd have hair.

The truth is there wasn't a universe, then there was a universe, so logically, some kind of god or prime mover must exist. And he hates you, so he made you bald. Why? I'm not sure.

I'd say it was something you did, but *even the current pope is bald*. If this is how God treats him, how do you think he'll treat you? In fact, there hasn't been a pope with a solid head of hair since Benedict XV in 1914. I mean, popes do everything God wants. They pray all the time. They keep their wee-wees in absolute mint condition. Ash Wednesday they go absolutely fucking apeshit. They don't even *vape*, for cryin' out loud! And still, God's given them nothing on top.

Sure, Pope Francis gets to live in his own tiny country, wear a nightgown all the time, has a car you can stand up in, and he can touch anything he wants in a museum, but all his friends are a bunch of guy virgins and he has parental control on his Internet. And for all of Pope Francis's sacrifices, he's just as bald as you. So unfair.

But maybe there's hope for him and for you. Not in this life, but the next one, which is why we ask:

Will I be bald in heaven?

Heaven with baldness is, again, ipso facto, not heaven. So, if heaven exists, it follows to reason you will have hair. If you can find proof of heaven then, you can now look at life as a twenty-to-seventy-year interlude of baldness that will be followed by an eternity with hair.

For me, this is the one reason to hold out hope, live my life ethically, and stop masturbating on airplanes. As much as it sucks to be bald, by withstanding it and even embracing it, we will be rewarded at our life's end by an everlasting return to hair.

That's why the kindest thing you can say to the widow of a bald man isn't "I'm sorry for your loss," or "He's in a better place," but "He has hair now." Please note that you can purchase a HE HAS HAIR NOW tombstone on verybald.com for just $2 (plus $28,000 shipping and handling).

Being bald, it is comforting to have a God to pray to and/or yell at. Plus, having a religion gets you holidays off work, while agnostics get nothing. Might as well just tell people you're *something* for the extra paid vacation. Fortunately, our society has many gods to choose from and most religions—except for Scientology—are free.

I'm sure you don't have time to test out every religion. Over the course of the past year, I prayed to several gods for hair and here is what I found:

God God, aka Jesus—nothing

Jewish God—nothing

Allah—zip, plus I accidentally left a $160 prayer rug on the bus

Zeus—nothing

Satan—nothing, told to leave mass

Chronos—head felt warm, but then nothing

Shiva—nothing, may not speak English

Thor—didn't work, but decent movie

Krishna—Krishnothing

Akal Purakh—nothing, but may not have been pronouncing it right

L. Ron Hubbard—N. Ot Hing

This experiment, I believe, proves beyond a shadow of a doubt that no god cares about bald people. Given the failure of such a small ask, I wouldn't recommend wasting your time requesting something huge like world peace.

However, there is one religion I believe does provide hope for the bald man, because it has a bald man at its center. I'm talking, of course, about Buddhism.

Technically, Buddha isn't a god because no one will let a bald guy have that much credit. He's more a kindred spirit, an obese hairless pal who makes you feel better about your own looks. "Hey," you think to yourself, "if he's that happy—and he's fatter and balder than I am—then why can't I also be happy?" I find a lot of comfort in the fact that Buddha's a gigantic sloppy mess, unlike Jesus with his long hair and tight bod, always up on his cross telling me to stop drinking.

One of the best parts of Buddhism is you don't have to memorize a huge book like the Bible and constantly quote it at other people. Instead, in Buddhism, there are just Four Noble Truths:

1. **The essence of life is suffering**—you already know this, you're bald.

2. **The cause of suffering is craving**—right, you crave hair and you can't have it.

3. **You can end suffering**—great, so you're gonna give me hair?

4. **The way to end suffering is to follow "The Eightfold Path"**—okay, this is already too many numbers and it sounds like you're not giving me hair.

The end to suffering is a process called "meditation." It's not like traditional praying, where a priest or rabbi keeps asking you to stand up, then tells you to sit down (I mean, just do all the standing parts at once, right?). Instead, in meditation you sit still, silently, legs crossed, for like twenty minutes and maybe only look at your phone twice that whole time.

In this process of meditation, your thoughts slow down. You realize that your so-called feelings are also just thoughts, and they fade away. After a while, you come to understand that even your identity, your name, your sense of self, are all just thoughts, and as those fade away, you become, in a real sense, nothing. And "nothing" can't be bald!

Then you snap out of your sacred nappy-poo, take a deep breath, look around, and realize you're bald again, which sends you back to rule number one, that life is suffering. But now you're outside of it and can see it for the illusion it really is, or something? Anyway, for less experienced Buddhists like myself, this process of "enlightenment" can take as long as a week.

Plus, as a practicing Buddhist, there are no services on weekends! You can watch NFL football! And college football! And if you get really into it and become a Buddhist monk, everyone shaves their heads, so no one will know whether you're actually bald, or just a shaved-head guy. And no one is more fun than Buddhist monks. Just ask . . . well, anyone besides Buddhist monks because they're not allowed to talk.

Best of all, your religion demands that your employer give you time to meditate at work! And they have to give you Buddhist holidays off! They can't make you work on Asala-Dharma Day! Or Bodhi Day! Or Obon! And if they won't give you Magha Puja off *and* Magha Puja Eve, you can just sue the shit out of them.

If shaving your head, wearing an orange robe, begging for alms, meditating constantly, and never talking again all sounds like too much of a commitment to you, another great option is converting to Islam, which only demands you drop everything and pray eight times a day.

However, mosques in America can understandably be paranoid

about outsiders, so to make your conversion convincing, you should be as radical as possible. This may have complications in other areas of your life. For one thing, you'll have to give up drinking and bacon, which explains why the entire Middle East is so angry. For another, your new imam may suspect that you are an FBI agent infiltrating their mosque to entrap innocent people. Thinking you're a mole, the imam may either feed you intentionally wrong information or recruit you to serve as a double agent.

Once the imam believes you're in the FBI, good luck convincing him otherwise. It's easier to just pretend he's right and say you're passing along his false information and let him figure out for himself later that you were playing both sides of this thing as an insane scam because you didn't want people to know you're bald.

To avoid any confusion, prior to even entering the mosque, you should probably walk directly into FBI headquarters, ask to speak to the director, and tell him you plan on becoming a radical Muslim and you absolutely refuse to give any information to the FBI. Ask for a notarized document stating you are not an FBI agent so the imam will trust you are just some bald guy who walked in off the street one day and decided he was a radical Muslim.

You may quickly wind up in prison. But good news, there's a whole Muslim scene in there.

Let's end with a prayer. Please bow your heads and ask for God's blessing, as we say:

The Bald Man's Prayer

Now I lay me down to sleep
I pray the Lord my hair to keep.
And if I bald before I wake
I pray the Lord others' hair please take.
As long as everyone's as miserable as me
I'll be as happy as a bald can be.

27

Toupee: Threepee

After the toupee had left it in shambles, I began slowly reassembling what remained of my life. I reshaved my head. I took my résumé off LinkedIn. My therapist and I entered couples counseling. I sent Bald Scott an Edible Arrangement that was returned, three weeks later, still arranged and uneaten. These small steps provided a bit of comfort, but I still sensed deep in my soul and on my head that the universe was unbalanced, and I had to take bigger action to make it right.

So it was that I found myself recently on Thai Airways Flight 383. I'd barely made it—right up to the last possible moment I couldn't decide if I was doing the right thing. Was it incredibly foolish to journey to Thailand to return the hair from my toupee to its rightful owner? Would it provide closure, or open a fresh wound? Would I be greeted with anger, confusion, indignation, glee, or something I couldn't imagine? In a nation of 70 million people, how would I even find whose hair it was?

I had no idea whether to pack for a

day or a decade, so I wore my standard uniform, the one that makes me welcome anywhere: MAGA hat, Colin Kaepernick jersey, cargo shorts, and Uggs.

As I arranged my four neck pillows for the flight, then fastened my barrel of beef jerky into its seat, I sensed a tremendous amount of tension. People were stealing looks at me, then glancing away, not wanting to be caught. I knew what would set their mind at ease.

I stood up from my seat, cleared my throat, and announced, "People of Thailand! I am going to your country to return the hair from my toupee to its original owner! I am not a sex tourist!"

There was stunned silence, and then the loudest round of applause I've ever heard, followed by a fourteen-hour flight where I received numerous private thank-you's. The three men who didn't applaud were clearly sex tourists.

Always eager to fully immerse myself in a new culture, I sat at the Bangkok Airport Starbucks and unrolled my map to think strategy. There was only one thing to do: I was going to door-to-door this bitch.

Eighteen Months Later

I had now begun to question my original mission. My initial euphoria had worn off and Thailand had grown exhausting. I ran out of money about six months into the trip and had to take work in a factory that made Old Navy jorts. My boss was completely unsympathetic to my pleas that sixteen hours a day, seven days a week, was inhumane. Significantly complicating things, she was only eight years old, and *her* boss was only six. It seemed like the further I got up the chain of command, the younger they were. I had once seen a baby eyeing me from behind a two-way mirror. He made some notes on a clipboard, then crawled away. I suspect he was running the whole operation.

They say he was the real-life inspiration for *The Boss Baby*, a claim I remain unable to verify.

By this time, I believed I'd met every single person in Bangkok. I'd become somewhat of a fixture in the city, and the locals had taken to calling me ใบหน้าสุนัขขนปลอม, which loosely translated I believe means "dog face with fake hair."

I had been gone so long my wife had apparently taken a lover, Keith. I couldn't blame her—why shouldn't she be happy? When I FaceTimed her, I would often see Keith in the background, naked except for an apron, making crepes. To this day, I still can't look at a naked man in an apron making crepes without bursting a blood vessel in my eye. My daughters were virtually unrecognizable to me. The six-year-old was driving and the baby had molted her plumage.

It had become clear that my journey to return my toupee hair to its rightful Thai owner—and thus symbolically free myself from the shackles of vanity—had gone awry and destroyed everything that was good in my life. "You don't know what you got until it's gone" applies equally to both *hair* and life. And while I could never get my hair back, my life was still up for grabs.

A voice inside me whispered, "If you love something, set it free," and, as at SalesCon, I knew in that moment what I had to do: I dashed up the sweatshop stairs, pushed open the fire door, ran onto the roof, and yanked off my toupee, again momentarily forgetting it was glued on. My head bleeding profusely for a second time, I tossed my hairpiece into the wind and watched as it rose poetically upward as if attempting to kiss a cloud, then sailed off like an obese duck.

As I watched it recede, a second voice then whispered, "Chase it! Chase the hair!" and I knew in that moment the first voice had been a complete charlatan, and I should only obey the second voice, which was much closer to how I sound in real life. I jumped off the balcony, fell eighty feet, and landed on a family of six riding a Vespa. I handed them a fistful of baht, commandeered the scooter, and gave chase to the toupee on the horizon.

The next three months were a blur as I scootered through Chachoengsao, Prasat Hin Khao, Mae Sot, Sukhothai, Lampang, Chiang Mai, and Chiang Rai; then the wind switched directions and I was forced to retrace my steps back to my starting point and then through Kanchanaburi, Ratchaburi, Phetchaburi, Prachuap Khiri Khan, Chumphon, and Phang Nga. I drove tirelessly day and night, blasted out of my mind on a Burmese mixture of methamphetamine and caffeine called ya ba, and stopping only every time there was a Wendy's or McDonald's.

Finally, depleted, exhausted, broke and broken, just as I was ready to say "Fuck it!" the toupee landed in Phuket. I dropped the scooter in the middle of the road, ran to the fallen hairpiece, grabbed it, and kissed it. (I even kinda Frenched it.) After the makeout sesh ended, I realized I was lying at someone's feet. I tilted my head upward and there was a small Thai man, who was either twenty-eight years old, or ninety-four, standing above me. The sides of his hair were long, the top shaved, and I knew in my heart that second: My toupee had come from his hair. The hairpiece knew its origin, and like a faithful pilgrim, or a migrating neotropical songbird, it had finally returned home.

The reunion was perhaps the most poignant thing I'd ever witnessed. The man clearly had never expected to see the hair again, and as much as I needed and loved that hair, he loved it more. We were just two men and a hairpiece locked into a perfect moment, neither of us wanting it to end.

Sobbing, he introduced himself as Lek, and explained that with a wife, a young family at home, and a completely worthless bachelor's degree in literature, he had had to sacrifice the one thing he loved the most: his hair. The toupee had apparently cursed us both. His wife had used the money he'd gotten from it to leave him for his father. Now, here he was talking to a bald man from half a world away, who also had a young family and a completely worthless bachelor's degree in literature. We were each facing a person who was somehow both stranger *and* soul mate.

We had each surrendered our hair in different ways, and in doing so, we had both destroyed our lives.

In that moment, I realized: The hair had never belonged to me. And as painful as it was for me to let it go, I knew Lek's joy was—to use a phrase—a hair more than my agony. Lek adjusted my toupee on his head and it fit perfectly. Somehow cosmically—he through addition, me through subtraction—we both seemed whole again. Lek and I embraced, and I felt feelings that only those who relinquish a toupee and those who receive a toupee can understand. The fact that I had paid $1,500 for it and he wasn't making a move for his wallet seemed, at that moment, a mere quibble.

I flashed my teeth at him and, fearful of getting bit, Lek recoiled. I giggled, then he realized: It was a smile. We balds are far more alike than we are different. Lek laughed, and smiled back. "A mess" doesn't even begin to describe the state of his dental care.

I'm not sure how long our hug lasted, but our communion was broken by a blast of warm air and a profound shudder. Monsoon season had arrived. The violent wind picked up and roared so loudly we had to scream bald pidgin to be heard. Torrents of water poured through the streets, scattering cars like so many children's toys. I held on to Lek as he clutched the toupee, but as we all know, human strength is nothing compared to that of Mother Nature. We were borne by an overwhelming current into the horror of a pounding, ferocious surf. Clinging to one another so deeply our nails drew blood, we swore to protect each other and both return home.

But alas, the monsoon had other plans. I was forced to drown Lek so I could survive. He wanted to live very badly, so it took several hours.

The toupee was last spotted in that big garbage island in the Pacific.

Coda

I retained a lock of the toupee to wear in a charm as a reminder of all I had suffered, but someone tore the chain off my neck at the Newark airport and ran off with it. I'm still unable to dislodge a balloon containing twelve pounds of ya ba from my large intestine. Lek's ex-wife and his father just had twins. "Uncle Keith" now lives in my pool house. He is bald.

28

So You Are Bald!

If you only take one thing away from this book, it should be this: Stop looking at the bald spot on your head. Don't examine it, poke it, project forward what it's going to be or backward to what it was. Do anything besides looking at your head—read a book, take a nap, pick your nose, touch a service dog even when they tell you not to. Literally anything is a better use of time than spending one more second focused on your head.

I stared at my head for twelve years and learned nothing. It never made me feel better. There was never any grand revelation about my hairline, or myself. There is no magic thought that will set you feeling right once and for all.

The harsh truth is: Your hair is gone. The same way you wouldn't dig up your dead grandmother and expect her to make you fudge, your hair ain't coming back. And if it does return, it will be some *Pet Sematary* ghoulish version of its former self.

If you have to look at the top of a head, look at mine:

I guarantee yours isn't worse than this—odds are, in fact, that it's better. But what you see and what I see looking

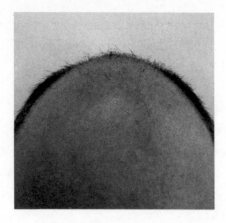

at this picture are probably two different things. You see a gross, ugly bald head whose hair abandoned it. I see the few heroic hairs that, in spite of everything, are still there.

Imagine the character, the determination, of these lone hairs. For years, they've watched as the world around them crumbled. Every hair they know has taken the easy way out, into a drain or onto a pillow. I spent more than a decade panicking about the ones that left, but now that those are gone, my feelings have shifted—I now appreciate the ones who faced incredible odds and stayed put.

I think of them as my "300." They are the soldiers of last resort, nobly defending a lost scalp against an impossible enemy—the final Spartans against the Persians of baldness.

Their bravery, their sacrifice, will never be forgotten so long as I am alive and balding. Day after day, they teach me the simplest and most profound lessons: Appreciate what you have. Love the one you're with. Let hairgones be hairgones.

And who knows? Maybe there's a cure right around the corner that will render this all irrelevant. I'd love nothing more than for this book to be pulped along with every copy of *Twilight*. Until then, I'm clinging just as tightly to my 300 as they're clinging to me.

But that doesn't mean I'm not prepared at all times. The second it's feasible to harvest hair from someone's body, I plan on shooting the hairiest man I can find with a tranquilizer gun, harvesting his follicles, and leaving him in a bathtub full of ice with a note that says, "This isn't that kidney thing."

In case that blissful moment arrives, I always keep a go-bag on me that will allow me to take a prisoner and steal their hair follicles. Now that you're not staring at your head, you have time to assemble one for yourself. Here is a checklist:

- Bag

- Medical-grade anesthesia. If you have major surgery and turn down the anesthesia, they will let you take it home.

- Barf bag (for victim).

- Raw steak, to quiet any guard dogs.

- Cheese, to quiet any guard hamsters.

- *The Shape of Water* DVD so you and your victim will have something to watch and discuss before or after.

- Grenades in case plan goes sideways.

- Size 3 shoes and bloody elf cap, to create fake trail and make it look like an elf did it.

- Boogie board—who says this can't be fun?

- Ziploc baggie for any tongues you have to cut off.

- Picture of yourself standing in giant pair of pants to show everyone how much weight you've lost.

- $800,000 cash.

- Two garbage cans full of ice—how else are you gonna fill the bathtub, dummy?

- This checklist.

- You!

Until the blessed day arrives when we can roam the countryside, tranquilizing people and commandeering their hair, there are many other real, simple steps we can take to improve the condition of all bald men in the world today.

Here is my Bald Bill of Rights:

Bald Bill of Rights

- Bald people should be allowed to DUI. Our lives are markedly worse than other people's, so we have plenty of reasons to drink. If everyone else gets .08, we should get at least a .25. I'd argue for a full 1.0, but I don't want to be unreasonable.

- When it comes to health insurance, baldness should be considered a preexisting condition and hair transplants should be as easy to get as abortions. Why not combine the two? If people don't want those babies, we'll take their stem cells.

- We should get to board first on planes. This would give all the bald people a minute to meet one another, because we know no one else will save us in case of a crash.

- Just as fines are doubled in construction zones, any crime against a bald man should be categorized as a hate crime and should incur twice the penalty, unless committed by a bald man, in which case it should be recategorized as a crime of passion and the penalty shall be half.

- A Bald Hall of Fame will be built directly on top of the Baseball Hall of Fame to show that being good at baldness is much harder than being good at baseball. Admission to the Bald Hall will get you admission to the baseball one, but not vice versa.

- A complete ban on all photography. This is self-explanatory and nonnegotiable.

- Barely anyone is using either Dakota. South Dakota will be renamed North Dakota. North Dakota will be renamed Baldakota and function as an independent homeland for the hairless, ruled by baldarchy. Any bald man shall be able to stake a claim of no less than five and no more than seven acres. Any woman who elects to live in Baldakota will be given a stipend of $8 million a year. A fifty-foot statue will be built in her likeness, or however she wants us to say she looks.

- In delis that give out tickets to patrons, we should never have to wait more than two spots. Bald people, upon proving baldness at a local DMV, should be issued a leather deli ticket with the permanent number of 3. While acknowledging that at any given time maybe two people have it worse than us and should go first, this will also minimize the time we have to spend being bald in delis, which for some reason is way worse than being bald everywhere else. Maybe because our heads kind of look like unsliced hams.

- As outlined earlier, the antibald bias in entertainment is currently the biggest problem facing the world today. Almost every bald character in a TV show or movie is either a drug kingpin, evil, or an alien who wants to take over the earth. What is the solution? The so-called Bechdel Test is used to measure male chauvinist bias in television, movies, and books. It posits that a feminist work needs to have at least two female characters who talk to each other about something besides a man. In a similar vein, I propose the "Baldskull Test." Every show, movie, or book should have at least two bald characters who talk to each another about something other than a person with hair, a drug deal, or destroying the earth. If a work doesn't pass the Baldskull Test, everyone involved in its creation will be buried alive.

- Bald people should each get to commit one murder without recourse. This would reduce discrimination and economic bias against us because people would have to wonder if we'd used our murder yet. Obviously, we shouldn't allow more than one murder, because that would open it up to abuse.

- Hair privilege will be officially acknowledged, and a delegation of haired leaders will present a formal apology to a delegation of balds at Yalta. The delegation of balds will reject the apology and formally tell the haired to go fuck themselves. The haired leaders will then publicly commit seppuku as restitution for "all the stuff we did." Thereafter, on January 1, 2020, every human being on earth (plus all animals) will legally be required to have their heads shaved so we can all start fresh on equal footing (or heading).

These are clearly sane, reasonable demands. But change takes time. Until that change comes, there are many things you, as a bald man, can do every day to improve the lives of bald people and our cause as a whole.

Buy Bald

Purchase only products manufactured by bald men by looking for the FBBB (For Bald by Bald) label. These products are handcrafted by bald artisans and a percentage of all profits will go to buying tiny horses for single bald men. All business will be transacted using the first decentralized cryptocurrency for the hairless, BaldCoin. We don't have a product line yet, but the first prototype is this comb designed specifically for bald men.

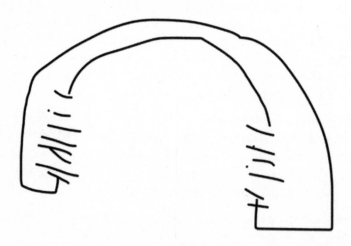

It gets the sides without scratching the top.
It will be made of endangered rhinoceros horn.

Donate Sperm

Wear a wig to the donation center and lie about being bald. This way we can secretly breed millions more bald men who will eventually help in our struggle. Even a couple ounces of sperm today could mean ten, twenty, or even a hundred bald men a century from now. Remember our mantra: Sperm Speaks Louder than Words.

Start Staging "Bald-Ins"

Imagine if thirty thousand bald men entered a Sears and refused to leave. They'd give us anything we want! It's worth just doing it now and figuring out what we want later.

Demand Baldchella

Let's get Pitbull, Billy Corgan, and Phil Collins to go to the desert, while we get high and dance with scantily clad bald guys while flying on Molly. No chicks allowed! Does life get any better?

Invest!

Take the money you save on haircuts and invest it in an index fund. Say you start at age twenty (let's assume $20 haircut and $1 tip, you cheap ass), you will have over $100,000 by the time you're sixty. That's not even counting the money you'll save on dates! Save now and dive back in when everyone's divorced and looking for their second husband!

Only Watch Pornography Where the Male Protagonist Is Bald

This would bring the free pornography business to its knees! (Or maybe it's already there, blowing someone.)*

Every Bald Man in the United States Should Join the NRA

The National Rifle Association has 4.5 million members. If all 40 million bald men joined, we would have a ten-to-one majority. We would instantly be a giant, well-armed bald militia, with unbelievable political clout. Yes, I'm suggesting we change the NRA to the Bald Rifle Association, or BRA. Finally, a BRA you can get into!

Imagine tens of millions of bald guys with submachine guns, running around open-carry states, using our right to bear arms to advance our right to bare heads! Imagine how safe you'd feel at schools, churches, and work, knowing there were heat-packin' baldies with their safeties off, ready to fire whenever they thought they saw anything slightly weird. Imagine being part of an angry, dangerous, heavily armed, untrained militia and getting group discounts at hotels because of it! Don't worry about it getting out of control—the only thing that can stop a bald guy with a gun is a balder guy with a gun!

This may sound crazy, but then again, they said Charles Manson was crazy. But he didn't have to do his own laundry, or cook his own meals, for over thirty years, so who's crazy now?

---

* Special "hello" to all my high school teachers! Thanks for the education! You didn't waste your lives at all!

29

(Kinda) Serious Conclusions

Let's imagine that one day you magically got your hair back—how would you be different? Would you suddenly know how to approach people and talk to them? Would you instantly have interesting things to say? Would you miraculously treat people in a way that they'd choose to be around you?

The answer to all those questions is probably going to be no. I'm betting you'd still be an insecure and bumbling bag of flesh and blood, but with hair.

Your problem isn't your hair—it's your personality. Your mind has tricked you into thinking your main problem is your lack of hair because it's the most noticeable thing about you. The truth is, you need to work on yourself, no matter what's happening in Swedish follicle labs, because at the end of the day, you'll still need to be at least a moderately good person to have a chance at anything you want, with hair or without.

Truth #1: Other people don't dislike you—*you* don't like you.

The main source of your agony isn't that other people won't date you or give you a job. It's projecting that if you were them, *you* wouldn't date you or give you a job.

The truth is, no one really cares about you or has opinions about you. They don't notice if you're bald, short, or on fire because everyone is worried *you're* looking at *them* and judging them as old, dumb, fat, or whatever. Just as you're agonizing over your head, they're spinning out over whatever they think their worst feature is. No one has the energy to even think about you because everyone is obsessed with themselves.

Baldness is a great teacher. Think about it. Who are you freaking out about? You. Who do you think other people are freaking out about? You? You really think they're fixated on some bald weirdo? Hell no. Their only concern is the person they're deluded into thinking other people are obsessed with, which is themselves.

And if everyone is trapped in this narcissism, why does *your* spiraling need to be some shameful secret? If the entire world's freaking out over their own crooked nose, webbed feet, or wonky eyes, it's something you have in common with everyone else—we're all panicking that we're flawed. That means you're normal! And by overlooking what's wrong with other people, you invite them to overlook your baldness. Mutual vulnerability can be a bridge.

Accepting others opens a path to accepting yourself, and accepting yourself opens a path to accepting others. Just as you can lock yourself into a negative spiral, you can also lock into a positive one.

I understand how bad hair loss makes things seem, especially if you're in your twenties and watching everyone hook up and get married while you can't even get a single date. I was there—every woman I knew just wanted to be friends. "Friends with benefits" hadn't even been invented back then. It wasn't until 2011 that people realized friends can also have sex. I basically spent all of 2001 through 2010 helping women repaint their apartments so they could get their security deposit back.

But once you hit your thirties, it all starts to slowly turn around, and you might not even have to change at all, because demographics are on your side.

You know how it feels like everyone's getting engaged? They are. Pretty soon, everyone worth being with will already be taken, so those left single will be in a mad scramble to wind up with someone, anyone.

You will not be exactly what she wants, and she may not be exactly what you want, but you both will be what you can have given that the older you get, the fewer the options. And maybe you lack chemistry, have nothing in common, are opposed politically, even hate each other, but you can still build a life. You will live under the same roof, have children, and raise them, and it will mostly feel annoying and weird. But over time, you will come to realize this friction, this anger, this constant fighting that leaves you both bereft and exhausted is, for lack of a better word, love.

And that's because you will *call* it love. And you will have made such an investment of time and energy that even if it doesn't feel genuine, there's no real sense picking away at it, because it only makes you both feel bad and there's no solution.

This has been going on since the beginning of time, all the way back to when Adam and Eve were each other's only options. And it will continue going on until the Yellowstone supervolcano explodes in about a month.

You need to question your longest-held beliefs and see if they still hold up under the extreme scrutiny necessitated by your elevated desperation. Who cares if someone loves you for *you*?

From birth, it has been hammered into us about the importance of love as the foundation of family, faith, and marriage. But do we really need love?

You are giving your partner a greater appreciation for what they don't have. So, later in life, after you've died, if they finally find six months of true love in a nursing home, can you imagine how much they'll appreciate it? What a wonderful gift you've given them!

When do you appreciate a piece of gum the most? After you just had a slice of cake? No! After you just puked fish! You are the fish puke that makes the gum taste so sweet! This isn't fantasy; it's real life.

Basically, be someone's compromise. It's fine.

The great thing about life is it catches up with everyone. The person who lectures you about money will lose theirs. The captain of the football team and homecoming queen will get fat. Friends who made fun of you for going bald may even go bald and then turn to *you* for advice (don't help them). You will see almost everyone you know get broken down by life and get their ass kicked and you know what? It's truly wonderful once you accept it. Your deterioration happened first via baldness, but your coping will happen first too. And once you come to terms with baldness, you get to watch a parade of others' suffering as you kick back in your easy chair and lose a couple more hairs to the antimacassar.

My journey through the different methods of hair replacement revealed to me the depth of the bald man's paradox, or "hairadox": Either baldness was responsible for everything wrong in my life and I'd wasted twenty years *not* having a toupee and now couldn't possibly make up for that lost time; or, now that I had hair, if my problems continued, they were never the fault of my hair at all, and I had wasted those twenty years worrying about my hair, when in reality it had no impact at all. Either way, you're wasting your time. It's all in your head, not on your head.

Remember all those strategies we learned so that baldness isn't the first thing people think about when they think about you? While learning them, we also made it so *baldness isn't the first thing you notice about yourself.* I don't care what other people think of you, the bald man; I care only what you, the bald man, think of *yourself.* It'd be great if someone falls in love with you, but even greater if you can at least enjoy your own company, so you're no longer spiraling down the drain of you. One awesome thing about being bald is that unless we're looking in a mirror, we never have to see ourselves. Our looks are mostly other people's problem!

Truth #2: You weren't that great with hair.

I was insecure before I lost my hair, and more insecure after. I was shy before and shy after. I was self-centered before and after. My problem was never hair. It was always insecurity. It was shyness. It was being self-centered.

We can cry all we want about baldness destroying our lives, but the truth is you probably weren't that awesome with hair. Are you Brad Pitt? Harry Styles? No? Then you were maybe, at best, just okay. You were always going to get old, your face was going to get destroyed, you'd lose your sex hormones, and by the age of fifty you were probably going to look like a sack of wet oatmeal with big old hips. At most, baldness robbed you of five good years, but knowing you, you would have wasted that entire time running software updates anyway.

If you were to get your hair back, as I found with my toupee, you'll instantly spot new things wrong with you. You will always have the same amount of worry; it will just be focused on different things. Your problem isn't hair. It's worry. Work on the worrying.

Hair makes your life easier, but that doesn't mean it's better or more meaningful. Any feat becomes greater if it's accomplished *in spite* of something. Obstacles are what give achievements value. Millions of people graduate from high school every year, but Malala Yousafzai did it in spite of the Taliban wanting to end her life simply for learning. That's why she's a heroine and every other high school student sucks.

Baldness certainly isn't the threat of getting shot in the face by the Taliban, but it ain't nothin' either. Eventually, you may find, as I did, that the opposition you get from baldness enhances your life instead of ruining it. Baldness is a weighted vest, and while it makes you suffer, it also makes you stronger. Your accomplishments shine brighter because they were achieved *while bald*.

Just as Ginger Rogers did everything Fred Astaire did "backwards and in high heels," you have to do everything people with hair have to do, but bald and in high heels. The degree of difficulty as you grow balder is exponential. Even seemingly routine tasks, from getting a job to getting a bartender's attention, are legitimate achievements for the bald man and should be treated as such.

But say you can't overcome hairlessness to achieve anything. What then? Well, if you fail at life, you've failed for a totally justifiable reason. You were defeated by the greatest opponent there is: baldness.

Do you remember who won the big fight at the end of *Rocky*? It wasn't Rocky, it was Apollo! The movie isn't about a great victory, it's about the fact that Rocky, a nobody, fought the best guy in the world and stayed in the ring. If, at the end of your life, you and baldness are both still standing, both bloody, having given it your all, clutching one another, and baldness whispers "Ain't gonna be no rematch," you've done the most heroic thing anyone can do—you've gone the distance against the greatest, the Muhammad Ali of physical detriments.

No one with hair knows what that's like, and few would have the determination to do it. You've taken blow after blow to your psyche, and just the fact that you're still even battling, like Rocky, means you won. And if you're screaming the name of a woman and she says she loves you—even if you're both Philly yuckos—so much the better.

Continuing to fight *is* the victory.

If your life isn't where you want it to be, cut yourself a break. It's hard going bald, and everything will take longer and be more difficult. And comfort yourself with the fact that people with hair fail all the time.

Remember I said this is the only book in the bookstore for bald people? Well, look around—you're probably in a giant self-help section for people with hair. (They're depressed.) There's a diet section.

(They're overweight.) There's a science fiction section. (They're nerds.) That so many people with hair are so miserable is a giant cause for joy. Those gloomy fat geeks can't fall back on our totally bulletproof excuse, which is that our life sucks because we're bald. They've been given everything the world has to offer and simply failed. They're the fucking losers, not us.

Truth #3: Baldness is a blessing. It woke you up. Told you, "Life isn't forever. Death's a-comin' and the world ain't fair!"

Maybe the hardest part of baldness is it serves as the first warning that everyone dies. Accepting baldness is, in part, accepting death. And death is terrifying. No more TV for a start, and all those people who tell you they want to pee on your grave get to pee on your grave. It's gonna be a freakin' grave pee-pee jamboree on my dead, bald head. And all I want is to live long enough to pee on their graves first.

A lot of people say they're going to pee on other people's graves, but I actually follow through. I pee on graves at least three times a week. It takes a lot of commitment and planning. Sometimes I'll hit a few in a day if Waze shows they're close. You have to ration your pee, but that's something you learn to do with experience and kegel exercises. All this will become easier once I complete beta testing on my new app, GravePee.

Death is the great equalizer. Everyone dies, and when they die, they go bald. We, unfortunately, experience that baldness while still alive.

As I've gotten older, I've come to terms with this, but not in the way you may think.

Every woman potentially contains within their genetic makeup a long-hidden baldness gene—that's why breeding is Russian roulette. You may not be bald, but a bald man's DNA could be lying dormant within her, watching, waiting for its next unwitting host.

I have two beautiful daughters. Thankfully, I'll never have to watch them grow bald. But part of me loves knowing they are booby-trapped.

Their looks, wit, and wiles will one day attract someone and honeypot that poor mark into unleashing my bald time bomb. It's the ultimate practical joke, creating another bald man from the great beyond. I like to believe if there is a heaven, I'll be looking down with a full head of hair and smiling at my panicking bald great-grandson. Hopefully, if he summons me to a séance, he won't be such a dick.

Truth #4: Baldness is a skill. The longer you're bald, the better you get at it and the easier it becomes.

Just like learning a musical instrument, the more you practice being bald, the easier it gets. Which means that this very moment, right now, is always the worst you will feel. It will only get better. If the goal is to be comfortable in your own skin, baldness gives you more skin to be comfortable in.

Unfortunately, not everyone goes bald, but fortunately, everyone gets old. First a couple of wrinkles, a little belly, veins in their hands, and soon they're totally freaking out. You, on the other hand, have spent twenty years with the weighted vest on, and when you finally get to take it off, you won't believe how light you feel. Everyone else is panicking, but you lost your hair decades ago. You get everything back on the B-side.

Bald ninety-year-olds are the happiest people you'll ever meet because they've put in their practice looking old. Past seventy, any guy's hair looks fake whether it's real or not. Time doesn't just level the playing field; it tilts it in our direction. I'm only forty-five and I'm already looking better than a lot of people I know with hair. Baldness bothers me less and less every day.

And if you're just going to end up being not worried about it later—and I can promise you this is true—that means it will *definitely* get better, which means *you don't need to worry about it now.* Just wait it out and in the meantime accept discomfort as a sucky but temporary part of life.

I could never have anticipated feeling this way ten or even five years ago, but maybe if someone had told me this then, I would have been spared all my self-inflicted agony. I can assure you that if *you* continue to worry, there is a 100 percent chance you will feel stupid for wasting your time later. You probably won't wish you had hair back—as I found with my toupee, that was a mixed bag—but you will definitely wish you had that time back.

I'm not going to lie and tell you it's easy. You'll always be able to find anger and resentment over being bald if you look. So you learn: It's stupid to look, so don't look. And that's what wisdom is: not doing what's stupid.

Truth #5: If baldness can make you hate yourself, then there's something wrong with the way you look at yourself to begin with.

I realize that for many people reading this, baldness isn't a joke. It's deadly serious. It makes your life worse minute by minute and tortures your existence.

I wrote this book because as I combed (sorry) message boards for information on medications, toupees, and transplants, I was struck by how many people baldness is driving to suicidal thoughts. I was one of them. And while I'm not a doctor (although my dad was, which kind of makes me a doctor), and you should get help from a (bald) professional, I hope this book can at least contribute, in a small way, to helping you feeling better and more normal.

That's why I've shared with you basically every intimate detail about myself, things even my family didn't know. I want you to have the information I didn't have. I want you to know you will gain perspective and it won't always seem so dire. I want you to be aware that you're part of a giant community and you're not suffering alone.

I also want money to buy a summer house.

This openness is, I hope, a new paradigm for baldness. If we can chip away at the secrecy that surrounds this thing, bring it out into the open, look at it, laugh at it, own it, and even enjoy it, maybe the shame and panic will drop away. Imagine how much power we will have, creating this visible support network! And again, if we all get shoulder-launched cruise missiles, the sky's the limit!

A saw doesn't care what you cut. A pencil doesn't care what you draw, whether it's masterful or dog shit. The same way, your mind doesn't care what you think. You can have anxiety and self-hatred or be the happiest, most positive person in the world.

Simply resolving not to kill yourself because of a few thousand stupid hairs is a small first step in making things better. It's true, what doesn't kill you only makes you stronger. Compared to baldness, every other obstacle in my life has been a breeze.

You should feel proud you are bravely facing something even John Wayne couldn't. When you're able to walk out of the house with your bald head showing to the world and feel no fear, no shame, no self-loathing, what can possibly harm you? Nothing. Except for spinal meningitis, brain aneurysms, and bears.

And even if things seem hopeless now, who and where you are today has no bearing on who and where you can be in a year, five years, or a decade.

To illustrate, a true story. In 2011, I was the final comedian to perform on the George Lopez talk show before it was canceled. As I was waiting to go on, the other two people backstage were—I'm not making this up—Paul Walker and Donald Trump. If you had looked at the three of us, me, Paul Walker, and Donald Trump, and said, "In eight years one of you will be the same, one of you will be dead, and one of you will be president of the United States," I would have said, "Oh my God, I'm going to die."

Then, after Paul Walker died, I would have looked at Donald Trump and said, "Oh my God, I'm going to be president."

Eight years later, Paul Walker is dead, Donald Trump is president, and I am a prominent member of the bald community. None of us can fit into the pants we wore that day (although it feels unfair to paint Paul Walker with that brush). But that's only eight years! Who knows where another eight could take us? Donald Trump could be bald, I could have a talk show, and Paul Walker could be the first dead president!

The emotions you feel today are not fated or permanent, they're temporary and will change. Maybe a pill or surgery will arrive that gives everyone lustrous hair. Maybe there will be an international nuclear incident that leaves everyone bald and you, being an experienced bald man, will wield an incredible amount of power. Maybe you'll cultivate some hobbies, meet some people, and turn that into some sex.

The future is wide open. Even though you're bald, there are so many great things still waiting to happen to you, things you'll appreciate even more because your baldness is a constant reminder of how bad things can be.

I had to work harder to get my wife, so I appreciate her more. I love my kids more because I know how hard I had to work to have kids.

It even helped me understand my father better after he passed away. My dad used to eat a slice of plain white bread every night with dinner. He explained it like this: "When I was on Guadalcanal during World War II, we didn't have any bread for months. All we ate was hardtack. Ever since I got home, plain bread tastes like cake. It actually tastes so good I don't need cake." This was fifty years after the war ended.

After baldness, imagine how small every other challenge will seem by comparison! For me, raising children is a breeze. My company laying off everyone is a joke. When Fox canceled my TV show, I said, "That's it? I thought you had bad news." I walk away from car accidents and don't even bother exchanging insurance. When my doctor told me that my cholesterol was "dangerously high," I told him he was "dangerously boring." I laugh in death's face! The worst has already happened, and I survived. And you can too.

People will take a "leap of faith" on God, where the proof is, let's say, dubious at best, but no leap of faith on themselves. Take a leap of faith on you. No one's sure about God, but you're here and you exist, and your life is in no way worth less because you're bald.

If anything, the bald man experiences a greater spectrum of feelings and therefore he *lives* more.

If I had hair, I don't know that I'd appreciate anything nearly enough or even at all. At the beginning of this book when I bragged I had a 1,500-square-foot house and $7,000 saved for retirement, you probably thought I was making a joke. Nope. If you had told me this was how I was going to wind up eighteen years ago when I started going bald, hated myself, and slept on a pile of my own dirty laundry, it would have seemed like a miracle. And it has been a miracle. What I have isn't a little, and it's not a lot, but I'm grateful for it. Whether I put the barriers in my own way or not, I still overcame them.

Everything is easy with hair. Everything is hard without it, and yet I've done as much as many people with hair, or even more!

I always dreamed of writing a book, but I never had a topic that felt interesting or important enough until I went bald. And now, my greatest agony helped make my dream come true. That's the power of the weighted vest.

So, here are my final thoughts, bald-to-bald: The worst has already happened. And if you have nothing to fear, that frees you up to live fearlessly. They can't take anything away from you that hasn't already been taken. Think—what is the very symbol of freedom in the USA? Why, it's an eagle, and that eagle is ... bald! Now you know the secret! Live that way!

For those of you who read this entire book in the bathroom, I sincerely hope you've enjoyed taking these shits as much as I've enjoyed being your companion for them. Good luck, and Godspeed!

And now, I set you free in the world.

Fly! Fly, bald man, fly! Soar! Live! Fly! Fly! Fly! No! You're headed directly for a windmill!!!

Acknowledgments

Hi! You've finished the book and now your reward is being forced to sit through a long, self-indulgent list of people you've never heard of thanked in the kind of flowery language no one ever uses in conversation.

First of all, I'd like to thank me. Without me, I could never have written this book. It was me who gave me the inspiration and, in my darkest times, me who picked me up so me could finish this manuscript so me could make some money so me and me family won't die.

I'd like to thank my literary agent, Erin Malone, who read the proposal for this book and thought, "We can make money off these hairless fucks," and helped my dream of publishing a book become a reality. I can't imagine another agent who would have covered up my drunkenness by lying that I'm a sex addict.

I'm deeply indebted to Luke Dempsey, my editor, who combines the ear of Mozart with the eye of Dalí. His faith and unflagging belief in this project uplifted and inspired me to finish throughout a difficult process. (← These are the only two sentences in the book he didn't want to change. Pretty fucking transparent, Luke.)

I'd like to thank my wife, Stephanie, and my kids and hope that in future therapy sessions they can discuss why they were only thanked after my agent and editor had already been thanked. They endured a year of me screaming "Can everyone shut up? I'm writing a book! Do you know how hard it is to write a book?!" even though most of the time I was locked in my study just reading espn.com and sleeping. Stephanie, you either actually love me or do such a great job pretending that I now buy it. I love you. Julia and Molly—thank God you are girls so you'll never go bald. Papa loves you. Now everyone go into another room and be quiet.

To my idol, Ayn Rand, who taught me that a book doesn't have to be good, it just has to be tens of thousands of words between two pieces of cardboard. Namaste.

I owe a tremendous debt to Craig Kilborn, who gave me my first TV writing job, and owe nothing to Craig Ferguson, who fired me from that job. Thanks to Mike Gibbons, who's always been a huge proponent of my writing, greatly damaging any respect I had for him.

Alec Sulkin and John Viener, who taught me that the best friendships are composed of a couple texts a month without any real insight as to what's going on with the other person. Thank you. I also owe a tremendous debt to Seth MacFarlane, who helped me buy my house by writing wiener jokes. I know you'll never read this, but thank you.

Friends from "The List"—I won't thank you individually because we are, after all, a secret email list. You know who you are, and perhaps even more important, others now know who they aren't.

My TV agent, David Stone—there's not a kinder or smarter person in this business. I still find it hard to believe he ran over a whale with his cigarette boat, but those nuns are credible and they saw what they saw.

I would not have all the money I have without Michael Cohen, my extraordinary accountant, who also just so happens to be bald. I guess we can both deduct our hair as a total loss.* My attorney, Karl Austen, I'm so grateful you're on my side, otherwise I'd be terrified of you. You are very courageous to take on hairless clients.

Thanks to Charlie Hankin for his beautiful illustrations of

---

* Very funny accounting joke.

things like a mustache being stuffed through a crotch. Gracias to Eli Green for shooting the cover photo that sent me into a three-month depression. Danke to my great friend Jared Hess for appearing in the self-defense section and actually letting me strangle him with a sweaty toupee. Merci to Christine Shaw for helping with photo clearance—this, quite literally, is the least I could do.

All the people who work cutting down trees and in the paper factory—your life hasn't been a waste, even though reading this, it seems like it maybe was.

Also, I'd just like to say to almost everyone I went to high school with, a huge "Fuck you."

To my mother and father, who told me, "Follow your dreams. You can do anything." You were wrong, so instead I published this book. Thank you for giving me every opportunity, and so sorry this was all I was able to do with it. Mom, I hope this book made you cry in a good way. I love you. My brother, Henry, who somehow has a full head of hair, you're so fucking lucky. You should really give me half.

My mother-in-law, Elaine Cline. You are a great grandmother and have proved your allegiance to the cause by once marrying a bald guy.

Special thanks to everyone at Fox who canceled my TV show *Making History*, which torpedoed my career so now I have to write a book like it's fucking 1850 or something.

Also, thank you to my doctor, Jordan Geller. Someday you'll be the one to tell me I'm dying. Until then, let's cherish the prostate exams by candlelight. I never could have written this if not for the help of my therapist, Alex Bloom. If you're incredibly fucked up mentally, you should talk to him.

John Voigtmann, Brian Frank, Mona Zutshi, Michael Bernard, and Chris Regan, thank you for keeping me as your token bald friend.

Travis Bowe and Kevin Biggins—thanks again for the rice. (We were driving back from Vegas hungover. I went to get gas and they ordered food for me. When I came back, they had gotten me rice instead of fries. What hungover guy wants rice? You idiots.)

Thank you to everyone at my publisher, HarperCollins, for all your assistance. Expecially Fred Wiemar, who helped with cpoy eidtng.

Then there are the important people. To the lady who works at the Pinkberry and didn't bat an eyelash even when I showed up three times in one day, thank you. Larry David, I'm just a worse version of you. To every woman who dated me—you were right, I wasn't the one. I'm very grateful to my Shakespeare professor, Edward Tayler, who said, "Graduate work isn't for you. Go to San Francisco and play your saxophone." (I was holding a saxophone at the time.)

Larry Bird, David Ortiz, and Steph Curry, it's incredible everything we've accomplished together.

I also owe a debt of gratitude to the famous people who wrote blurbs for the book. Basically, I only wrote this book so if it's successful I can blurb other books. That way if I'm in a bookstore, I'll know if I'll like a book because I'll see a quote on the back from me saying I liked it.

There are others whose names I'm sure I forgot because ultimately they aren't that important to me. If you weren't named and feel you should have been, you should be completely offended. Use this as an opportunity to never talk to me again.

Most of all, I'd like to thank all my fellow bald dickheads out there who keep waking up and persevering day after day, God knows why.

About the Author

The so-called "bard of baldness," Julius Sharpe was raised in Lexington, Massachusetts, home to the American Revolution and then nothing since. In high school, he was a national debate champion—in other words, a complete fucking loser. He went to Columbia University and majored in astrophysics, until a professor who'd won a Nobel Prize in the field called him an idiot. Sharpe then switched to English, which was way easier.

After graduating, Julius pursued stand-up comedy, destroying all his parents' dreams. He performed on *The Late Late Show*, *Jimmy Kimmel Live!*, and *Lopez Tonight*. In fifteen years of stand-up, he made a total of almost eleven thousand dollars. Concurrently, he held several temp jobs in IT. If he ever worked for you or your company, he knows he was terrible and would like to apologize. He's not giving the money back, though.

Julius's life changed for the better when a pile of jokes he submitted via email miraculously got him hired on *The Late Late Show with Craig Kilborn*. He has since written for *The Cleveland Show*, the Academy Awards, *Family Guy*, and *The Grinder*. He created *Making History* for Fox, which the *New York Times* called "funny and endearing" and "borderline gross."

Literally nothing else interesting has ever happened to him.

Julius has a great life, a loving family, a wonderful wife, and two amazing children. But he would trade it all for hair.

This is hopefully his last book.